DIABETES AND HYPERTENSION

A fatal attraction explained

~

BRYAN WILLIAMS

BSc, MD, FRCP
Professor of Medicine, University of Leicester

PUBLISHING
INITIATIVES
BOOKS

Doral House • 2(b) Manor Road • Beckenham • Kent • BR3 5LE

A note about the author

Bryan Williams graduated in medicine at St. Mary's Hospital Medical School, University of London in 1983. His initial medical appointments were in London, followed by training in medicine and nephrology in Leicester and the University of Colorado Health Sciences Center, Denver, USA. In 1991, he was awarded a British Heart Foundation Research Fellowship and, in 1993, became Senior Lecturer in Medicine at the University of Leicester, and an Honorary Consultant Physician at the Leicester Royal Infirmary where his principal clinical interests are vascular disease and hypertension. He was appointed Professor of Medicine in 1996. In 1993, the BUPA Medical Foundation awarded Dr Williams the title 'Doctor of the Year' in recognition of his research into diabetic vascular disease and, in 1994, he was awarded the Linacre Medal by the Royal College of Physicians in recognition of his research work. He has published numerous papers on the cellular mechanisms of vascular injury with particular reference to diabetes. He is currently a member of the British Hypertension Society, the British Renal Association, the European Society of Hypertension and the International Society of Hypertension, and is a fellow of the American Council for High Blood Pressure Research. Dr Williams is a member of the Association of Physicians, UK and Ireland, and is a fellow of the Royal College of Physicians, London.

ACKNOWLEDGEMENTS

*I would like to acknowledge the expert
secretarial assistance of Sarah Holden and her
help in preparing this book.*

Printed by the Lowfield Printing Company Ltd, Dartford, Kent, UK.

*First Published 1996.
Reprinted 1997.*

ISBN

1 873839 38 3

Further copies of *Diabetes and hypertension* may be obtained from Pi books, a division of Publishing Initiatives (Europe) Ltd. This publication reflects the view and experience of the author and not necessarily those of Pfizer Ltd or Publishing Initiatives (Europe) Ltd.

Foreword

My introduction to diabetes was through hypertension. As a very minor satellite in the Pickering blood pressure constellation of the early 1950s, I was given the task of testing the assertion that not only was hypertension more common in people with diabetes, but that this increased prevalence extended to the non-diabetic members of their families. The mysterious link was already suspected and some constitutional, familial or genetic mechanism inferred.

One problem in constructing the study was the question of exactly what was hypertension and, it then transpired, what exactly was diabetes? Pickering *et al* had come to the view that hypertension was not so much a quality as an extreme of the quantity, arterial pressure; that the cause was 'multifactorial'; and that the associated cardiovascular risk rose (though not necessarily linearly) across the whole pressure range. Platt and his colleagues did not agree. The aetiological ding-dong which ensued was a classic of the century.

The history of non-insulin dependent diabetes (NIDDM) has had strong similarities. It is one of the quirks of history that the qualitative (bimodal) hypothesis for NIDDM has been most strongly protagonised by Dr Peter Bennet, originally out of the Platt stable while I, with diminishing fervour, have defended the quantitative (unimodal, continuous distribution) corner.

What has all of this to do with Bryan Williams' masterly mid-1990s tour of the same horizon of diabetes and hypertension? At least we now have formal definitions for them, thanks to the WHO consensus. Of course the defining values are challenged. As arbitrary cut-offs, laid on continuous variables, so they always will be. The big question is at what point we should intervene, and how. Raised arterial pressure is so much more damaging to people with diabetes than those without that the case for earlier intervention is strong - but unfortunately not yet evidence-based.

It really does look as if the range of arterial pressure is about the same in the person with insulin dependent diabetes (IDDM) as in the person without diabetes until renal disease accelerates its rise. But it is a range, and it may be those at the top of that normal range who are liable to diabetic kidney disease, microalbuminuria, clinical proteinuria and declining glomerular function. And it may be the genetic/constitutional factors that place them high in the pressure range which also mediate their renal susceptibility.

In NIDDM, arterial pressures are high at diagnosis but these people are older and fatter, many of them already with early evidence of retinal and renal microvascular disease. The plot thickens as evidence accrues that relative insulin resistance plays a part in the liability to nephropathy as well.

However the fatal attraction is to be explained, hypertension and diabetes make bad companions and important practical medicine. Professor Williams is to be congratulated on his comprehensive review of the epidemiology, the mechanisms and the available antihypertensive therapies with their indications in diabetes. We come right up to date with consideration of angiotensin receptor blockade as a potential future therapy, but not at the expense of a thoughtful evaluation of the great array of agents now available.

I cannot totally escape a sense of personal responsibility, however, when I read Professor Williams' comment that *'It is remarkable that no large, population-based, randomised trials of antihypertensive therapy have been conducted in diabetic patients'*. That highly undesirable state of affairs is likely to be redressed over the next few years, but clinicians must not wait. The circumstantial evidence for potential benefit is so strong that vigorous and effective therapy in the hypertensive diabetic patient is as much an imperative as blood glucose control. This book will help us greatly in tackling this task.

Harry Keen, Emeritus Professor of Human Metabolism
and Honorary Consultant Physician, Guy's Hospital Campus
United Medical and Dental School (UMDS)

Contents

List of abbreviations 11

Introduction 12

Chapter 1 - Epidemiology of hypertension in patients with diabetes 15

Introduction 16

Prevalence of hypertension in IDDM and NIDDM 16

Influence of age on blood pressure in diabetes 18

Influence of gender on blood pressure in diabetes 19

Influence of ethnicity on blood pressure in diabetes 19

Conclusions 20

References 20

Summary points 21

Chapter 2 - The pathogenesis of hypertension in diabetes mellitus 23

Introduction 24

The pathogenesis of hypertension in IDDM 24

Microalbuminuria and blood pressure in diabetic patients 25

Ambulatory blood pressure monitoring 26

The role of sodium retention in the hypertension of IDDM 28

Renin-angiotensin system and hypertension in IDDM 29

Changes in vascular reactivity in hypertensive IDDM patients ... 30

Endothelial dysfunction and the hypertension of IDDM 31

The pathogenesis of hypertension in NIDDM 32

Sodium and hypertension in NIDDM 33

Obesity, NIDDM and hypertension 33

Microalbuminuria and blood pressure in NIDDM 36

Contents

Other causes of hypertension in diabetic patients 36

Isolated systolic hypertension 37

Renal artery stenosis in diabetes mellitus 38

Malignant hypertension 39

Conclusions 39

References 39

Summary points 41

Chapter 3 - Diabetes and hypertension: a fatal attraction 43

Introduction 44

'Diabetes mellitus is a vascular disease' 45

Macrovascular disease 47

Microvascular disease 51

Diabetic retinopathy 54

Diabetic neuropathy 56

Diabetic nephropathy 57

Hypertension and mortality in diabetes mellitus 58

Diabetes and hypertension, a 'fatal attraction' 58

References 59

Summary points 60

Chapter 4 - Diabetes mellitus: a conspiracy of cardiovascular risk factors 61

Introduction 62

What is insulin resistance? 62

The basis of insulin resistance 64

Cardiovascular risk-factor clustering associated with diabetes mellitus: the role of insulin resistance 65

Contents

Insulin resistance and cardiovascular
  risk-factor clustering 70

Insulin resistance and cardiovascular disease
  in 'Westernised' Asian communities 71

'Diabetes mellitus is a conspiracy of cardiovascular
  risk factors' 72

References 73

Summary points 74

Chapter 5 - Diabetic nephropathy, microalbuminuria and proteinuria 75

Introduction 76

Definition and epidemiology of diabetic nephropathy 76

How many diabetic subjects get diabetic nephropathy? 79

Why don't all diabetic patients get nephropathy? 81

What is microalbuminuria? 82

How is microalbuminuria measured? 83

Recommendations for screening and monitoring of
  microalbuminuria 83

Risk factors for the development of microalbuminuria 85

The significance of microalbuminuria in IDDM 86

The significance of microalbuminuria in NIDDM 86

Microalbuminuria is not just a marker of renal disease 87

Microalbuminuria, proteinuria and diabetic microvascular disease 87

Macroalbuminuria, proteinuria and diabetic macrovascular disease ... 90

The significance of microalbuminuria in the non-diabetic population 92

Why does microalbuminuria predict generalised vascular disease? 93

Microalbuminuria: an important surrogate for accelerated
  vascular injury 95

Contents

References 95

Summary points 97

Chapter 6 - Evaluation of the diabetic patient with hypertension 99

The problem of defining hypertension in diabetic patients 100

Guidelines on the guidelines 101

Towards a consensus from available guidelines 102

Blood pressure measurement 104

Clinical evaluation of the hypertensive diabetic patient 104

Key points in medical history 105

Drug therapies that may elevate blood pressure 105

Physical examination of the hypertensive diabetic patient 106

Physical and simple laboratory findings suggesting secondary
     hypertension 107

Investigation of diabetic subjects with hypertension 108

Further investigations 109

References 109

Summary points 110

Chapter 7 - The treatment of hypertension in diabetic patients 111

Goals of therapy 112

Antihypertensive therapy: treatment goals 112

Non-pharmacological treatment of hypertension in diabetic subjects 112

Non-pharmacological treatment of hypertension 113

Who will benefit from non-pharmacological treatment? 114

Summary of non-pharmacological treatment 115

Contents

Pharmacological treatment of hypertension in diabetic subjects 115

Ideal drug therapy for hypertension in diabetic subjects 115

Thiazide diuretics 116

Mode of action 116

Benefits of thiazide therapy 116

Potential adverse effects of thiazide diuretics in diabetic subjects
with hypertension 117

Indapamide 118

Conclusion 118

Beta-adrenergic blockers 118

Mode of action 118

Benefits of beta-blocker therapy 119

Potential adverse effects of beta-blocker therapy in diabetic
subjects with hypertension 119

Conclusions 120

Alpha₁-adrenergic blockers 120

Mode of action 120

Benefits of alpha₁-adrenergic blockers 120

Potential adverse effects of alpha₁-adrenergic blockers in diabetic
subjects with hypertension 122

Conclusions 122

Calcium antagonists 122

Mode of action 122

Benefits of calcium antagonists 123

Potential adverse effects of calcium antagonists in
diabetic subjects with hypertension 124

Conclusion 125

Contents

Angiotensin converting enzyme (ACE) inhibitors 125

Benefits of ACE inhibitors 125

Potential adverse effects of ACE inhibitors in diabetic patients with hypertension 127

Conclusion 128

Other antihypertensive therapies 128

Sympatholytic agents 128

Direct vasodilators 128

Angiotensin-II receptor antagonists 129

Initiating drug therapy in hypertensive diabetic subjects 130

Follow-up of diabetic patients with hypertension 131

Drug therapy selection 131

Combination therapy 131

Drug therapy selection in specific clinical situations 134

Hypertensive IDDM subjects with no microalbuminuria or proteinuria 134

Hypertensive NIDDM subjects with no microalbuminuria or proteinuria 134

Isolated systolic hypertension in diabetic subjects 135

Diabetic autonomic neuropathy and supine hypertension with orthostatic hypotension 136

Impotence in diabetic subjects with hypertension 137

Left ventricular hypertrophy in diabetic subjects with hypertension ... 137

Left ventricular dysfunction and congestive heart failure in diabetic patients with hypertension 138

Ischaemic heart disease and post-myocardial infarction in diabetic patients with hypertension 138

Renal artery stenosis in diabetic subjects with hypertension 138

Contents

Ethnic differences in response to antihypertensive therapy 139

Diabetic nephropathy, microalbuminuria and proteinuria 139

Calcium antagonists in hypertensive diabetic subjects with
microalbuminuria and proteinuria 140

Is it important to lower urinary protein excretion in diabetic
subjects? 141

IDDM patients with hypertension and microalbuminuria or
proteinuria 142

NIDDM patients with hypertension and microalbuminuria
and proteinuria 144

Normotensive IDDM patients with microalbuminuria 146

Normotensive NIDDM patients with microalbuminuria 147

*The underdiagnosis and undertreatment
of hypertension in diabetes* 147

Concluding remarks 149

References 150

Index 153

List of abbreviations

ACE	angiotensin converting enzyme
ACR	albumin:creatinine ratio
AI	angiotensin-I
AII	angiotensin-II
BHS	British Hypertension Society
BMI	body mass index
CT	computerised tomography
CV	cardiovascular
CHD	coronary heart disease
CCF	congestive cardiac failure
DBP	diastolic blood pressure
DCCT	Diabetes Control and Complications Trial
ECG	electrocardiogram
GFR	glomular filtration rate
HDL	high-density lipoprotein
IDDM	insulin-dependent diabetes mellitus
ISH	isolated systolic hypertension
LDL	low-density lipoprotein
Lp(a)	lipoprotein (a)
LVH	left ventricular hypertrophy
MRFIT	Multiple Risk-Factor Intervention Trial
NIDDM	non-insulin-dependent diabetes mellitus
PAI-1	plasminogen activator inhibitor-1
PDGF	platelet-derived growth factor
RAS	renin-angiotensin system
SBP	systolic blood pressure
UAER	urinary albumin excretion rate
WHO	World Health Organisation
WHR	waist:hip ratio
UKPDS	United Kingdom Prospective Diabetes Study
UKWP	United Kingdom Working Party

Introduction

Hypertension is both a common and a potentially devastating complication of diabetes mellitus, a true fatal attraction. Independent of diabetes, hypertension is established as a major risk factor for the premature development of cardiovascular (CV) disease and CV death. When associated with diabetes, the potency of hypertension as a CV risk factor is further enhanced.

Identifying and treating hypertension has always been an important component of diabetic care. Nevertheless, for obvious reasons, achieving good glycaemic control has been the main focus of the clinical management of diabetic subjects for many years. The results of the recent Diabetes Control and Complications Trial (DCCT) has justified this approach and has confirmed the efficacy of good glycaemic control in delaying the development of microvascular disease, i.e. retinopathy and nephropathy, in patients with insulin-dependent diabetes.

It is noteworthy, however, that by far the most common form of diabetes is non-insulin dependent, and the major cause of premature morbidity and mortality in these subjects is macrovascular disease. To date, there is little evidence to suggest that strict glycaemic control in subjects with non-insulin-dependent diabetes (NIDDM) will postpone their myocardial infarction, their stroke or their death. In contrast, hypertension is very common in these individuals and there is ample evidence confirming a strong link between an elevated blood pressure and the development of macrovascular disease. Moreover, there is also an impressive body of data confirming that the effective treatment of hypertension can reduce CV risk. Although most of the patients studied in the trials that have confirmed the efficacy of antihypertensive therapy have been non-diabetic, there is no reason to believe that the proven benefits of antihypertensive therapy will be any less in diabetic subjects. On the contrary, because the CV risk associated with hypertension is greatly magnified by the co-existence of additional CV risk factors, it is reasonable to conclude that the benefits of antihypertensive therapy may be even greater in diabetic subjects.

In preparing this book, I have attempted to highlight areas of clinical consensus and the many controversies and uncertainties that confront the clinician when managing hypertension in diabetic subjects. In important areas where the lack of clinical data has frustrated my attempts to be precise and dogmatic, I have drawn on my own clinical experience and that of others in attempting to be pragmatic. After all, even though the benefits of some forms of antihypertensive therapy in some clinical situations remain unproven, for the hypertensive diabetic patient the stakes are high and the consequences of no therapy have become abundantly clear.

Thus, in the management of patients with diabetes, there is no reason why the long established obsessional approach to glycaemic control should not be matched by an equally enthusiastic approach to the management of hypertension and other CV risk factors. It is indeed conceivable that the latter may ultimately be proven to be more important in reducing CV morbidity and mortality than the former. In this regard, the fact that hypertension in a significant proportion of diabetic subjects remains undetected, untreated or inadequately treated is a major cause for concern and represents an enormous opportunity missed. This opportunity to minimise the CV risk experienced by diabetic subjects has been further enhanced by recent exciting developments in CV risk factor screening, individualised risk stratification and our expanding therapeutic armamentaria. These new developments are at last being put into clearer clinical perspective by recently published and soon to emerge clinical trials. The need, the desire and the opportunity to improve further the management of hypertension in all patients with diabetes have never been greater.

Chapter One

EPIDEMIOLOGY OF HYPERTENSION IN PATIENTS WITH DIABETES

Introduction

Diabetes and hypertension are common conditions in Western societies. They frequently co-exist, more often than can be accounted for by chance. It is often stated that hypertension is at least twice as common in people with diabetes than among the non-diabetic population. This statement is not necessarily wrong, it simply hides the complexity of the truth. The relationship between arterial blood pressure and diabetes mellitus is much more intriguing and defies description in a single sentence. Many reports have attempted to define the epidemiology of hypertension in diabetic patients. Over the years, these studies have produced conflicting results and in many cases have confused rather than clarified the situation. Many such studies failed to control adequately for the diverse factors known to influence blood pressure levels independently. Some studies have used inadequate or historical controls, others have failed to allow for important contributory factors such as age, gender, ethnicity, degree of obesity, type of diabetes or presence of renal disease. It is also noteworthy that the definition of hypertension is arbitrary and varies from study to study in accordance with the guidelines of the day. Fortunately, more recent studies have endeavoured to take account of these issues and in so doing have produced more consistent data that perhaps more reliably define the fascinating and important epidemiological relationship between blood pressure and diabetes.

Prevalence of hypertension in insulin-dependent diabetes mellitus (IDDM) and non-insulin-dependent diabetes mellitus (NIDDM)

The frequency of hypertension was recently examined by the London Diabetes Hypertension Study Group in a large sample of patients (5,842) with both IDDM and NIDDM aged 18-69 years[1]. The blood pressure readings in all patients were taken in standardised conditions. For the whole sample, systolic blood pressure (SBP) and diastolic blood pressure (DBP) were significantly and positively correlated with both age and body mass index (BMI). Consequently, the unadjusted SBP and DBP are higher in NIDDM patients when compared to IDDM, because the former tend to be older and more obese. Nevertheless, even when the blood pressure values are adjusted to take account of differences in age and BMI, SBP and DBP are still significantly higher in NIDDM than in IDDM subjects. This was convincingly demonstrated by analysis of data from the Joslin Clinic in Boston, US, which collected information on diabetic patients from 1964-65. When the data from diabetic men and women were compared to the non-diabetic population of the US, an excess prevalence of hypertension was evident in those with diabetes for all age groups[2].

Table 1 - The frequency of treated and untreated hypertension (defined by WHO criteria: BP ≥160/≥95 mmHg) in IDDM and NIDDM patients stratified by type of diabetes, age and gender.

IDDM				NIDDM			
<40 years		≥40 years		<55 years		≥55 years	
Male	Female	Male	Female	Male	Female	Male	Female
6%	6%	29%	25%	29%	31%	43%	52%

Moreover, as the duration of diabetes increased, there was a gradual divergence between the age-adjusted blood pressures of the diabetic and non-diabetic populations.

The frequency of hypertension in any study population is dependent on the criteria used to define hypertension. The Diabetes and Hypertension Study Group used the arbitrary World Health Organisation (WHO) definition of hypertension, i.e. SBP ≥160 mmHg or DBP ≥95 mmHg (see Table 1)[1]. Using these values, hypertension was uncommon (6%) in IDDM patients under 40 years old with no gender differences. In older IDDM patients (≥40 years), hypertension was much more common (29% of men and 25% of women). In NIDDM patients, the frequency of hypertension was much higher, more common in females and markedly influenced by age (particularly SBP). In younger NIDDM patients (<55 years), the frequency of hypertension was 25% in males and 31% in females. In older NIDDM patients (≥55 years), it had risen to 43% in males and 52% in females. The pattern of these results was not influenced by differences in the distribution of patients with proteinuria, as the prevalence of proteinuria was equivalent (5%) in IDDM and NIDDM patients.

A similarly high prevalence of hypertension has also been reported in newly diagnosed NIDDM patients (aged 25-65 years) in the United Kingdom Prospective Diabetes Study (UKPDS). Of the initial 3,648 recruited in the UKPDS, 39% were hypertensive and, once again, more women (46%) than men (35%) were affected (see Table 2)[3]. This suggests that almost 50% of NIDDM patients are hypertensive at diagnosis, which is much higher than an expected prevalence rate of about 30% in the similarly-aged non-diabetic population. When stratified for age, it shows the apparent effect ageing has on the prevalence of hypertension in men and women with NIDDM (see Table 3)[3].

Table 2 - Prevalence of hypertension in newly diagnosed NIDDM patients recruited to the UKPDS study. Hypertension is defined as receiving antihypertensive therapy or a mean blood pressure of ≥160/≥90 mmHg two and nine months after the diagnosis of diabetes.

	Men	Women
Number studied	2136	1512
Age (years)	52±9	53±9
On therapy	14%	24%
Not on therapy (BP≥160/≥95)	21%	22%
Total hypertensive	35%	46%

Table 3 - The prevalence of hypertension (BP: ≥160/≥90 mmHg) in the UKPDS study of 3,648 NIDDM patients stratified according to age and gender.

Males					
Age (years)	25-34	35-44	45-54	55-64	Total
Hypertensive (%)	13.5	28.0	33.8	40.2	34.7
Females					
Age (years)	25-34	35-44	45-54	55-64	Total
Hypertension (%)	16.6	36.5	43.9	53.4	46.5

Influence of age on blood pressure in diabetes

Ageing is associated with an increase in blood pressure in both the diabetic and non-diabetic population. This is most noticeable for SBP. These changes are thought to reflect ageing of the larger vessels which lose their elasticity, resulting in a loss of vascular compliance. This reduction in vascular compliance favours a widening of pulse pressure and an elevation of SBP. This explains the frequent development of isolated systolic hypertension in elderly patients. As indicated above (Tables 1 and 3), ageing has a marked effect on the prevalence of hypertension in both IDDM and NIDDM patients. It is also apparent that the effects of ageing on blood pressure are much more pronounced in people who are diabetic when compared to those who are non-diabetic. This latter observation may reflect accelerated ageing, greater injury and/or increased fibrosis of the larger vessels in the diabetic patient. In this regard, it is an old notion that the blood vessels of the diabetic patient function as though they are at least 10 years older than the patient.

Influence of gender on blood pressure in diabetes

The role of gender in determining the prevalence of hypertension in patients with diabetes has been the subject of conflicting data. Some studies have suggested a higher prevalence of hypertension in women, with others showing no difference. In the more recent studies cited above, the overall prevalence of hypertension was about the same by gender except for the older patients with NIDDM in whom hypertension was clearly more common in women, thus implying that the age-related rise in blood pressure was steeper in female diabetic patients. It is interesting to compare these gender effects with those observed in the non-diabetic population. In the non-diabetic, normotensive population, the age-related rise in blood pressure during adulthood is also steeper in women, so that by their seventh decade women have SBP levels that equal or exceed those of men. In hypertensive, non-diabetic women this 'crossover' occurs earlier with the prevalence of hypertension eventually reaching, and then surpassing, that of men at 45-55 years of age. It is clear, however, that in diabetic patients, this 'crossover' occurs even more prematurely so that the blood pressures of women with diabetes exceed those of men with diabetes at least a decade earlier than would otherwise be expected. This observation suggests that diabetes negates the CV advantages normally experienced by women in their premenopausal years.

Influence of ethnicity on blood pressure in diabetes

In addition to age, gender, BMI and the presence of renal disease, another potential influence on blood pressure is ethnicity. In the US, multiple studies have concluded that hypertension is more prevalent, more severe and often associated with more target organ damage in both non-diabetic and diabetic Afro-Caribbean people. In the UKPDS study of newly diagnosed NIDDM patients, the highest mean blood pressures were also found in Afro-Caribbean people. The lowest blood pressures were observed in Asian people, with the whites occupying the middle ground. The differences in blood pressure between white and Asian people were not significant after adjusting for age and BMI. Another UK study from Birmingham also found a higher prevalence of hypertension in Afro-Caribbean patients with diabetes (48.9%) when compared to white people (37.5%) and Asian people (35.4%)[4]. It thus seems that hypertension is indeed more common in Afro-Caribbean people with diabetes. Moreover, target organ injury also appears to be more common and more pronounced in Afro-Caribbean people for any given level of blood pressure.

Conclusions

Hypertension is very common in patients with diabetes. In IDDM, it is relatively uncommon in younger patients, but becomes much more prevalent with ageing. There is also a very powerful influence of diabetic nephropathy on the prevalence of hypertension in IDDM which is discussed in more detail in Chapters 2 and 5. In NIDDM, even using the high threshold values of 160/95 mmHg for the diagnosis of hypertension, it is remarkably common, particularly in women, with up to 50% of patients being affected.

There appears to be an important ethnic influence on the prevalence of hypertension, with hypertension being more common in Afro-Caribbean people when compared to white or Asian people. Diabetes also appears to accelerate the effects of ageing on blood pressure in both IDDM and NIDDM patients so that isolated systolic hypertension becomes common at a relatively early age in diabetic patients when compared to the non-diabetic population.

REFERENCES

1. Fuller JH, Stevens LK, Diabetes Hypertension Study Group. Prevalence of hypertension among diabetic patients and its relation to vascular risk. *J Hum Hypertens* 1991; **5**: 237-43.

2. Krolewski AS, Warram JH, Cupples A, Gorman CK, Szabo AJ, Christlieb AR. Hypertension, orthostatic hypotension and the microvascular complications of diabetes. *J Chron Dis* 1985; **38**: 319-26.

3. The Hypertension in Diabetes Study Group. Hypertension in Diabetes Study (HDS): I. Prevalence of hypertension in newly presenting type 2 diabetic patients and the association with risk factors for cardiovascular and diabetic complications. *J Hypertens* 1993; **11**: 309-17.

4. Pacy PJ, Dodson PM, Beevers M, Fletcher RF, Taylor KG. Prevalence of hypertension in White, Black and Asian diabetics in a district hospital diabetic clinic. *Diabetic Med* 1985; **2**: 125-30.

CHAPTER 1 - SUMMARY POINTS

- Hypertension is more common in diabetic patients than in the non-diabetic population.
- Hypertension ($\geq$160/90 mmHg) exists in at least 6% of young IDDM patients. The prevalence would be much higher at a lower threshold (e.g. $\geq$140/90).
- Hypertension is remarkably common in NIDDM patients, affecting approximately 50%.
- Hypertension is more common in Afro-Caribbean patients with diabetes.
- The age-related rise in blood pressure is exaggerated in diabetic patients, which probably reflects accelerated ageing of the diabetic vasculature.
- Isolated systolic hypertension is particularly common in diabetic patients.

Chapter Two

THE PATHOGENESIS OF HYPERTENSION IN DIABETES MELLITUS

Introduction

The prevalence, time course and pathogenesis of hypertension differ markedly between patients with IDDM and those with NIDDM. In patients with IDDM, blood pressure is usually normal at presentation and commonly remains normal during the first 10-15 years of diabetes. The development of hypertension in IDDM is closely linked to the development of nephropathy. In contrast, hypertension is frequently apparent at diagnosis of NIDDM. The increase in blood pressure is generally correlated with increased obesity, decreased physical activity and the more advanced age that is characteristic of NIDDM patients. The role of nephropathy in the pathogenesis of hypertension in NIDDM is less clearly defined, but, unlike IDDM, nephropathy is not the major factor in the high prevalence of hypertension in NIDDM patients.

The pathogenesis of hypertension in IDDM

The development of hypertension in IDDM is strongly related to the development of clinical evidence of diabetic nephropathy. Diabetic nephropathy is usually defined clinically when urinary protein excretion is increased and proteinuria is detectable on a standard urine dipstick test. This usually indicates the excretion of more than 300 mg of albumin over 24 hours. More sensitive methods for detecting proteinuria have enabled the increase in proteinuria associated with nephropathy to be detected much earlier, during the microalbuminuric phase of the disease process.

Microalbuminuria is defined as an increase in urinary albumin excretion above normal, i.e. >30 mg per 24 hours, but less than that required to produce a positive stick test using a standard urine dipstick analysis, i.e. <30 mg per 24 hours (see Chapter 5 for a more detailed account of microalbuminuria). It is now clear that once the urinary albumin excretion rate is persistently elevated into the microalbuminuric range in IDDM patients, the patient's blood pressure begins to rise. Thus, in IDDM patients, the transition from normoalbuminuria to microalbuminuria is associated with a progressive year-on-year rise in blood pressure; this has been approximated to an annual rise in mean blood pressure of 3-4 mmHg. This progressive increase in blood pressure is paralleled by a progressive rise in urinary albumin excretion so that, after a few years, the patient is clearly hypertensive and has developed proteinuria. At this stage, the patient is labelled as having developed diabetic nephropathy. Thus, the prevalence of hypertension in IDDM is strongly influenced by the presence of renal disease as indicated by microalbuminuria or proteinuria. Before the development of an increase in albumin excretion rate, the prevalence of hypertension in IDDM patients is equivalent to that of the non-diabetic background population (see Table 4)[1]. Once microalbuminuria has become established, blood pressure progressively increases. Even using the liberal WHO criteria for hypertension (≥160/95), 30% of patients with IDDM and microalbuminuria are hypertensive, and 60% of patients with IDDM and proteinuria are hypertensive. If more stringent thresholds for the definition of hypertension are applied, i.e. 140/90, then at least 50% of IDDM patients with microalbuminuria and almost all of those with proteinuria could be expected to be hypertensive.

Table 4 - The prevalence of hypertension (%) in IDDM patients aged 30-39 years. Hypertension is defined as receiving antihypertensive medication or a blood pressure of ≥160/95 mmHg.

	Women	Men
Background population	1.7	3.1
Normoalbuminuria	2.2	3.1
Microalbuminuria	26.7	15.4
Proteinuria	86.5	77.8

Microalbuminuria and blood pressure in diabetic patients
The relationship between blood pressure and the development of microalbuminuria is an intriguing one. Mathieson examined this relationship prospectively in 205 IDDM patients over a six-year period[2]. During that time, 15 patients developed persistent microalbuminuria. Analysis of blood pressure records demonstrate that following the onset of persistent microalbuminuria, there was a progressive year-on-year rise in both systolic and diastolic blood pressure in the microalbuminuric patients. There was no such year-on-year rise in those patients who retained a normal albumin excretion rate (Figure 1)[2]. Although for a majority of microalbuminuric patients the blood pressure may remain within the arbitrarily defined 'normal range' for many years, there is no doubt that for the individual, the blood pressure is high and continues its inexorable rise. The mechanism for this progressive rise in blood pressure is undefined; however, histological studies of kidneys from patients with persistent microalbuminuria demonstrate that early morphological lesions are already developing within the glomerulus. Moreover, in patients with persistent microalbuminuria, significant fluid retention is already developing and there is an increase in exchangeable sodium (see below) correlating with the rise in arterial blood pressure. These observations suggest that in IDDM patients, the rise in blood pressure, which parallels the onset of microalbuminuria, relates to subtle early injury to the kidney and fluid retention.

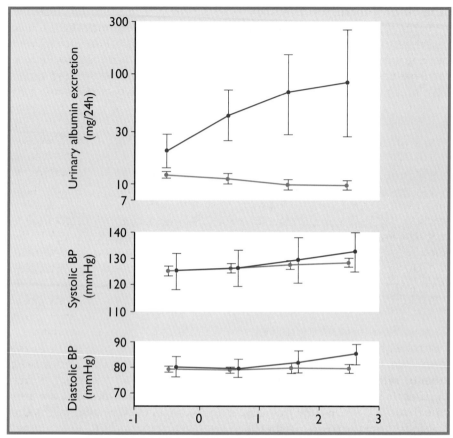

Figure 1 - Urinary albumin excretion and blood pressure (BP) in relation to duration of persistent microalbuminuria (•) (15 patients) compared with 190 patients who continued with normoalbuminuria (•). Mean and 95% confidence interval are given.

Essential hypertension can of course develop in IDDM patients in the absence of nephropathy. The prevalence of essential hypertension appears to be similar to that in the general population. Raised blood pressure due to essential hypertension in IDDM patients may be distinguished from that due to nephropathy as, for any given level of blood pressure, urinary albumin excretion is less and renal function is usually unimpaired in essential hypertension.

Ambulatory blood pressure monitoring
The use of 24-hour ambulatory blood pressure monitoring in IDDM patients has highlighted additional abnormalities in blood pressure regulation in IDDM patients with microalbuminuria or proteinuria. In non-diabetic normotensive subjects and the majority of patients with essential hypertension,

mean blood pressure declines by approximately 20% from day to night. Reduction in this diurnal variation of blood pressure is known to occur in hypertension associated with chronic renal disease, and is associated with the development of target organ damage in hypertensive individuals. Disturbances in diurnal variation of blood pressure have also been reported in IDDM patients with microalbuminuria[3]. This observation is very important because it suggests that in microalbuminuric IDDM patients, even though their 'office' blood pressure may remain within the normal range for some time, their overall 24-hour blood pressure burden is increased. This may explain why some patients with microalbuminuria often have early clinical evidence of target organ damage, such as left ventricular hypertrophy, despite seemingly normal 'office' blood pressures. Ambulatory monitoring is not widely available, nor is it practical as a routine assessment in general practice. Nevertheless, the fact that the presence of persistent microalbuminuria or proteinuria may itself be indicative of an increase in 24-hour blood pressure load, implies that microalbuminuria could become a surrogate for an abnormal ambulatory blood pressure profile and an increased blood pressure burden.

In addition to the progressive rise in blood pressure heralded by the onset of microalbuminuria, and the abnormal 24-hour diurnal variation of blood pressure, there is further evidence of abnormal blood pressure regulation in patients with microalbuminuric diabetes. It has been demonstrated that the normal increase in blood pressure during exercise is exaggerated in diabetic patients with microalbuminuria when compared to those without[4]. Taken together, it is clear that the seemingly normal 'office' blood pressure of a patient with microalbuminuric diabetes hides a spectrum of abnormalities in blood pressure regulation (Table 5).

Table 5 - Recognised abnormalities in blood pressure regulation in diabetic patients with microalbuminuria, when compared to those with a normal protein excretion rate.

- Progressive rise in blood pressure once microalbuminuria is established (annual mean blood pressure rise of 3-4 mmHg).
- Disturbed diurnal variation in blood pressure and a blunting of the normal nocturnal fall in blood pressure leading to an increased blood pressure load.
- Exaggerated response to pressor stimuli.
- Development of these changes despite a seemingly normal 'office' blood pressure.

The role of sodium retention in the hypertension of IDDM

Numerous studies point to an important role for sodium in the pathogenesis of hypertension associated with both IDDM and NIDDM. The fact that the total exchangeable sodium pool is expanded in diabetes has been recognised for many years, and in the 1960s prompted Conn to suggest that diabetes is a form of hyperaldosteronism. In both IDDM and NIDDM, the exchangeable body sodium pool is expanded even in normotensive individuals by approximately 10%, independent of age, obesity, sex or the presence of complications.

In hypertensive diabetic patients, the degree of sodium excess is at least a further 10% greater and is directly proportional to the blood pressure (see Figures 2[5] and 3[6]). This increase in exchangeable sodium relates to a relative impairment of sodium excretion as the excretion of a sodium load is blunted in diabetic patients. In effect, diabetes is a sodium-retaining state. Although sodium retention is prominent, blood and plasma volume are normal, if not contracted, in diabetes. Thus the expanded sodium pool implies that the extravascular space is enlarged (interstitial oedema), in contrast with essential hypertension where the sodium pool is usually normal.

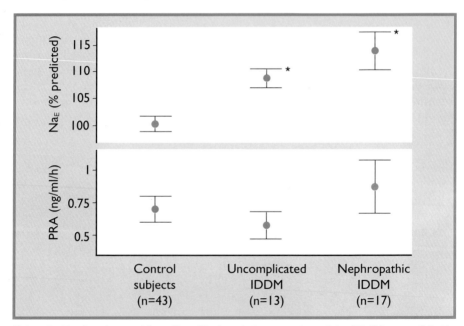

Figure 2 - Total exchangeable sodium (Na_E) and plasma renin activity (PRA) in non-diabetic control subjects, insulin-dependent diabetic patients without clinically detectable complications and insulin-dependent patients with overt (Albustix-positive) nephropathy. Means ± SEM. *$p < 0.005$ vs. controls.

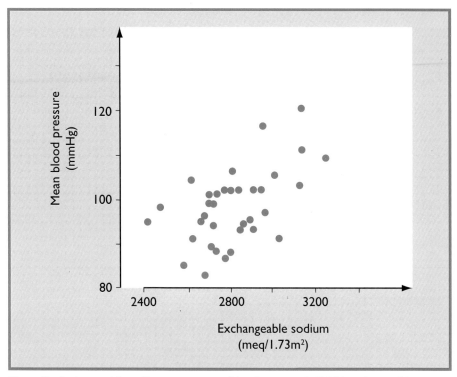

Figure 3 - Exchangeable sodium versus mean blood pressure in IDDM patients with elevated urinary albumin excretion (30-300 mg/24 h, i.e. incipient diabetic nephropathy); r=0.54, p<0.001.

Renin-angiotensin system and hypertension in IDDM

There has been much confusion and controversy over the potential role of the renin-angiotensin system (RAS) in the hypertension of diabetes. In normotensive IDDM patients without microalbuminuria or proteinuria, there appears to be an inverse relationship between plasma renin concentration/activity and blood pressure or urinary sodium. Thus in these patients the RAS is appropriately suppressed. In contrast, in IDDM patients with nephropathy, there appears to be no such suppression of the RAS despite even more marked sodium retention and higher levels of blood pressure. Thus, just as in other forms of renal disease, the nephropathic IDDM patient (microalbuminuira or proteinuria) experiences marked sodium retention and an inappropriately elevated activity of the RAS, which together contribute to the elevation of blood pressure (see Figure 2)[5].

The plasma concentrations of the various components of the RAS have been measured in IDDM patients with and without nephropathy, and compared to

Table 6 - Renin-angiotensin-aldosterone system in IDDM patients and normal control subjects.

Plasma concentrations	Normal control subjects (n=15)	Urinary albumin excretion <30 mg/24h (n=19)	Urinary albumin excretion 30-300 mg/24h (n=36)	Urinary albumin excretion >300 mg/24h (n=18)
Inactive renin (µIU/ml)	129 (49-231)	134 (51-308)	232 (26-790)	356 (87-1204)
Active renin (µIU/ml)	33 (12-64)	33 (7-93)	35 (8-76)	36 (10-76)
Renin substrate (ngAI/ml)	1509 (1066-2098)	1489 (1077-1879)	1455 (1066-1846)	1664 (1167-2390)
Angiotensin-I (pg/ml)	30 (14-93)	23 (8-78)	20 (11-42)	22 (8-38)
Converting enzyme (UCE)	25 (15-46)	29 (15-60)	33 (19-56)	30 (15-62)
Angiotensin-II (pg/ml)	14 (4-28)	7 (2-18)	6 (2-15)	5 (2-9)
Aldosterone (ng/100ml)	4.8 (1-11)	3.8 (1-14)	3.8 (1-15)	2.9 (1-7)

non-diabetic control subjects. It is notable that angiotensin-I and angiotensin-II plasma levels are lower in IDDM when compared to controls, whereas angiotensin converting enzyme (ACE) levels appear to increase as proteinuria develops (Table 6)[6].

Attempts have been made to quantify other humoral factors that may influence sodium exchange and blood pressure in IDDM patients. In patients with non-uraemic, metabolically well-controlled IDDM, plasma aldosterone, adrenaline and noradrenaline levels are all normal, if not low. Atrial natriuretic peptide levels are normal or slightly increased, the latter perhaps representing a compensatory response to sodium retention. These changes in the levels of aldosterone and atrial natriuretic peptide do not appear to be of primary importance in explaining the aforementioned sodium expansion and hypertension.

Changes in vascular reactivity in hypertensive IDDM patients
Although plasma angiotensin-II and catecholamine levels tend to be normal, if not low, in IDDM patients when compared to non-diabetic people, CV responsiveness to these agents is often exaggerated. This increased vascular

sensitivity, particularly to catecholamines, appears to occur independently of age, duration of diabetes or type of diabetic therapy. It is likely to arise via two possible mechanisms:

1. **Sodium retention** increases vascular responsiveness to pressor agents. The use of diuretics to reduce exchangeable sodium in diabetic patients has been shown to normalise the augmented vascular response of IDDM patients to catecholamines and promote a fall in blood pressure.

2. **Hypertension** results in remodelling of the resistance vessels leading to an increase in the vascular wall:lumen ratio. These changes in vessel structure are accompanied by an increase in sensitivity to pressor agents. It is possible that these pathophysiological changes act together to enhance vascular sensitivity to pressor stimuli and thereby contribute to the hypertension of diabetes.

Endothelial dysfunction and the hypertension of IDDM

The vascular endothelium plays an important role in regulating blood flow and blood pressure. Under normal conditions, the endothelium continuously liberates nitric oxide which acts as a potent vasodilator. Inhibition of this basal production of nitric oxide is associated with a rise in systemic blood pressure suggesting that nitric oxide plays an important role in the regulation of basal vascular tone and blood pressure. In addition to vasodilators, the endothelium also releases endothelins; these are extremely potent vasoconstrictors which may also play a role in blood pressure regulation. The endothelium also produces various prostaglandins, such as the vasoconstrictor PGH_2 or the vasodilator prostacyclin. Studies, in the main, support the hypothesis that the normal balance of endothelial function is disturbed in IDDM patients leading to a substantial defect in vasodilatation[7]. This may relate to a relative decrease in nitric oxide synthesis and/or an increase in vasoconstrictor prostaglandin synthesis. This reduced capacity of the vessels of IDDM patients to dilate could contribute to the development of hypertension in these patients. The mechanisms underlying the diabetes-induced development of endothelial dysfunction are not clear. However, there is ample evidence to suggest that the high glucose concentrations that constantly bathe the endothelium of diabetic patients, have the capacity to disturb endothelial function profoundly. Moreover, elevated lipid levels are also encountered in IDDM and NIDDM patients, and hyperlipidaemia has also been shown to influence endothelial function and perhaps contribute to the development of hypertension[8].

The pathogenesis of hypertension in NIDDM

Hypertension is very common in NIDDM and is present in at least 50% of patients at the time of diagnosis of NIDDM. The hypertension of NIDDM shares some common mechanisms with the hypertension of IDDM. However, important differences in the pathogenesis of hypertension exist between the two classifications of diabetes. Unlike IDDM, most hypertension in NIDDM is not explained by the development of nephropathy, the characteristics of NIDDM hypertension being more in keeping with co-existent essential hypertension. Unlike IDDM patients, in whom the blood pressure is often normal for at least 10 years after diagnosis, blood pressure is often raised at the time of diagnosis of NIDDM. In fact, blood pressure is also elevated in patients with impaired glucose tolerance prior to the diagnosis of NIDDM.

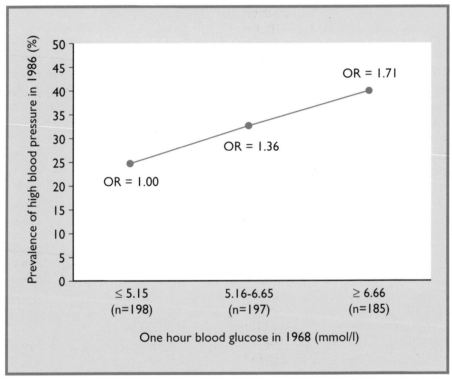

Figure 4 - Odds ratios (OR) for hypertension after 18 years in 580 initially normotensive (BP<160/95 mmHg) men according to tertiles of blood glucose value one hour after a standard oral glucose load. The odds ratios are adjusted for age, body mass index, alcohol intake, and initial systolic and diastolic BP. No intervention was implemented during the time of follow-up.

Blood pressure and blood glucose concentration appear to be related variables, and glucose tolerance is a powerful predictor of future hypertension. This was confirmed in a long-term follow-up of middle-aged men in Finland[9]. The normotensive men all had their glucose tolerance assessed in 1968 and then re-examined in 1986. The men with the higher blood glucose values following a standard oral glucose load in 1968, had a higher prevalence of hypertension in 1986 (see Figure 4)[9]. There is a tendency for hypertension to co-segregate with diabetes in families, perhaps reflecting a common genetic predisposition to both hypertension and glucose intolerance. There is little doubt that in young children and adults, blood pressure and glucose tolerance are closely related variables with potent powers of cross-prediction. In other words, if you are hypertensive you are more likely to be glucose intolerant and *vice versa*. Moreover, if you have hypertension or diabetes, there appears to be an increased likelihood that your parents or siblings were or will be hypertensive and/or diabetic. This supports the aforementioned hypothesis that similar genetic and/or environmental factors may contribute to both conditions.

The precise mechanisms explaining this association are not entirely clear. Obesity is common in both NIDDM and hypertension, and this is an important factor in the development of hypertension in NIDDM patients. Moreover, ageing is associated with higher blood pressures and NIDDM patients tend to be older. Nevertheless, these factors alone do not adequately explain the high prevalence of hypertension in NIDDM, and some of the factors highlighted above for IDDM patients, in particular sodium retention and perhaps also endothelial dysfunction, may also be involved in the hypertension of NIDDM.

Sodium and hypertension in NIDDM

Exchangeable sodium is increased in NIDDM patients who are normotensive and free of clinically apparent vascular complications. There is a strong, significant and positive association between exchangeable sodium and SBP in NIDDM patients (Figure 5)[5], suggesting that NIDDM hypertension is at least in part sodium-dependent. Just like the situation in IDDM patients, this increase in exchangeable sodium in NIDDM is not associated with any evidence of volume expansion in the hypertensive patients free of renal disease. Plasma renin is also suppressed in normotensive and hypertensive NIDDM patients free of long-term complications.

Obesity, NIDDM and hypertension

It is often stated that the high prevalence of hypertension in NIDDM patients is attributable to obesity. More than 80% of individuals with NIDDM are obese, and the prevalence of both NIDDM and hypertension increase with increasing body mass index. There is no doubt that obesity contributes very

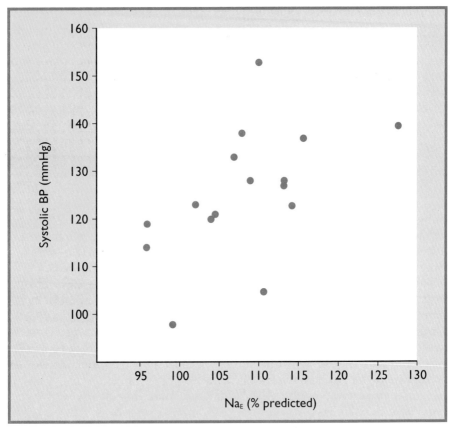

Figure 5 - The relationship between systolic blood pressure and exchangeable sodium (Na$_E$) in patients with non-insulin-dependent diabetes, who were free of long-term complications of their disease. r=0.53, P<0.05.

significantly to the high prevalence of hypertension in NIDDM. Nevertheless, it is also clear that when the epidemiological data is adjusted to account for the impact of obesity on blood pressure, there is still a considerable excess of hypertension in NIDDM patients. Thus, obesity is the most powerful factor influencing the relationship between NIDDM and hypertension, and acts to magnify this association, but is insufficient to explain it fully.

It has been recognised for a number of years that being overweight profoundly influences blood pressure. From general population data it has been calculated that in a normal individual, a gain in weight of 3 kg is associated with an increase in mean blood pressure of 1 mmHg, regardless of age or gender. Moreover, weight reduction is usually associated with a fall in blood pressure.

The explanation for the development of hypertension in obese patients is still being debated. It has been possible to demonstrate changes in circulatory haemodynamics, and it has been suggested that these changes are at least in part due to increased sympathetic nervous system activity. More recently, it has been suggested that insulin resistance and hyperinsulinaemia may contribute to the increase in sympathetic nervous system activity and also to the development of hypertension.

Circulatory haemodynamics and obesity
Characteristic changes in haemodynamics occur in obese individuals. These changes include an increase in cardiac output and a fall in peripheral vascular resistance. However, the fall in peripheral vascular resistance does not fully compensate for the increase in cardiac output, thus pressure rises.

Insulin resistance and hyperinsulinaemia
Insulin resistance is defined as a defect in the insulin-stimulated uptake of glucose. This defect is usually selective, involving some insulin actions in some tissues but not others. Decreased insulin-stimulated glucose uptake by skeletal muscle is a characteristic defect in NIDDM. This leads to reduced efficiency of post-prandial glucose disposal and a compensatory increase in the release of insulin. Thus insulin resistance is associated with hyperinsulinaemia. A similar defect in glucose disposal has been documented to occur naturally with ageing; it also occurs in obese individuals without NIDDM and in both obese and lean patients with essential hypertension. As these conditions are often associated, it has been proposed that insulin resistance and/or the resulting hyperinsulinaemia might actually be responsible for the development of hypertension in essential hypertension, in ageing people, in obese people and in NIDDM[10].

Mechanisms proposed to account for the link between insulin resistance/ hyperinsulinaemia and hypertension
Three hypothetical mechanisms have been proposed to explain how high insulin levels could potentially give rise to an elevated blood pressure.

1. *Sodium retention due to the antinatriuretic properties of insulin*

   There is little doubt that acute elevations of plasma insulin can reduce renal sodium excretion, and thus lead to sodium retention. However, it is still disputed whether chronic hyperinsulinaemia leads to a sustained antinatriuresis.

2. *Insulin-stimulated sympathetic nervous system activation*

   Supraphysiological levels of insulin stimulate the sympathetic nervous system in 'normal man' in a dose-dependent manner. It has been suggested that hyperinsulinaemia could lead to a chronic increase in sympathetic nervous system activity and thereby increase sodium retention, peripheral vascular resistance and cardiac output, and thereby elevate blood pressure.

3. *Insulin-induced vascular growth*

The third mechanism proposes an action of insulin to stimulate vascular growth. Laboratory studies have shown that insulin is a powerful growth factor for vascular cells. This observation has been used by some to suggest that high circulating levels of insulin could potentially influence vascular growth, promote the development of vascular hypertrophy and influence peripheral vascular resistance and blood pressure. This latter suggestion is the most speculative and least plausible.

It must be stressed that these proposed links between insulin resistance and hypertension remain a hypotheses and are unproven. It is my opinion that insulin resistance and hyperinsulinaemia play little or no role in the patho-genesis of hypertension and that they represent two commonly associated manifestations of another, as yet unknown, abnormality. Nevertheless, insulin resistance is common in hypertension and is associated with charac-teristic changes in body fat distribution and dyslipidaemia, all of which are very important and contribute to the CV risk attributed to hypertension in diabetic and non-diabetic patients[11]. This concept is discussed in detail in Chapter 4.

Microalbuminuria and blood pressure in NIDDM

The relationship between microalbuminuria and blood pressure is less well defined than in IDDM patients (see above), and is confounded by the fact that hypertension is frequently established in NIDDM patients before the diagno-sis of diabetes or nephropathy. Nevertheless, microalbuminuric NIDDM patients usually have higher blood pressures than normoalbuminuric NIDDM patients. Moreover, microalbuminuric NIDDM patients also exhibit abnor-malities in blood pressure regulation, similar to those observed in micro-albuminuric IDDM patients, i.e. a blunted nocturnal fall in blood pressure so that the overall 24-hour blood pressure burden is increased[12].

Other causes of hypertension in diabetic patients

Diabetic patients are also prone to develop hypertension due to causes other than those intrinsically related to their disease. Essential hypertension may occur by chance, renovascular disease is perhaps more common and isolated systolic hypertension certainly occurs earlier. There are also those rarer situ-ations in which diabetes and hypertension can co-exist as secondary conse-quences, such as thyrotoxicosis, phaeochromocytoma, Cushing's syndrome

Table 7 - An outline classification of the various mechanisms potentially accounting for the development of hypertension in IDDM and NIDDM patients.	
Insulin-dependent diabetes mellitus (IDDM)	Diabetic nephropathy (most common) Essential hypertension Isolated systolic hypertension (with ageing)
Non-insulin-dependent diabetes mellitus (NIDDM)	Essential hypertension (most common) Hypertension related to obesity Diabetic nephropathy Isolated systolic hypertension (with ageing)
Endocrine causes for a combination of diabetes and hypertension	Thyrotoxicosis Cushing's syndrome Phaeochromocytoma Acromegaly Primary hyperaldosteronism (diabetes v. uncommon) Some synthetic oestrogen/progestogens
Other causes of hypertension in IDDM or NIDDM patients	Renovascular disease Other chronic renal disease Aortic coarctation

and acromegaly. Other causes of secondary hypertension must also be considered, for example aortic coarctation, non-diabetic renal diseases etc. A classification of hypertension in diabetes mellitus is shown in Table 7.

Isolated systolic hypertension

Isolated systolic hypertension (SBP >160 mmHg, DBP normal i.e. <90 mmHg) commonly develops in the non-diabetic population with ageing. This reflects reduced compliance of the larger blood vessels as they age. Isolated systolic hypertension develops much earlier in diabetic patients and is common in middle-aged NIDDM patients. This appears to be due to acceleration of the vascular ageing process in diabetic patients.

Renal artery stenosis in diabetes mellitus

Unilateral or bilateral renal artery stenosis can lead to the development of severe hypertension. In the most cases (except in children and the very young) the renal artery stenosis is due to atheromatous vascular disease. The propensity of patients with long-standing diabetes to develop accelerated vascular disease suggests that renovascular abnormalities could be more common in the diabetic population. Nevertheless, the prevalence of renovascular disease in patients with diabetes is still unclear. This is because no thoroughly validated non-invasive screening methods to detect renal artery disease have been applied to patients with diabetes.

One of the largest analyses in the world literature refers to data from over 5,000 autopsies and reported on the incidence of anatomical renal artery stenosis (i.e. stenosis >50% of a renal vessel lumen). The study showed that anatomical renal artery stenosis does appear to be more common in patients with diabetes at autopsy (Table 8)[13], but the overall frequency of renal artery stenosis was low in all groups. Bilateral renal artery disease appeared to be more common in diabetic patients when compared to those without diabetes. The problem with autopsy data is that they cannot provide information about the functional significance of the vascular stenosis. In living patients with diabetes, the risk of renal artery stenosis has only been investigated in selected and small groups of patients. Some of these studies have suggested a higher prevalence of renal artery stenosis in diabetic patients with hypertension when compared to normotensive controls, but other studies have reported no difference. The available evidence would suggest that renal artery disease may occur with increased frequency in diabetic patients, reflecting the accelerated development of vascular disease in general. It is most unlikely to be the cause of hypertension in young IDDM patients and will more commonly be encountered in NIDDM patients. Identification of patients with renal artery stenosis is important because it has implications with regard to antihypertensive medication and is a potentially remediable cause of hypertension and renal insufficiency in these patients.

Table 8 - The calculated frequencies of renal artery stenosis detected at autopsy in over 5,000 patients with or without diabetes and hypertension.		
	Diabetes mellitus	
Hypertension	**Yes**	**No**
Yes	10.1%	6.1%
No	4.4%	1.0%

Malignant hypertension

There is little information available specifically relating to malignant or 'accelerated' hypertension in patients with diabetes. Clinical experience and anecdotal reports suggest that malignant hypertension is no more common in diabetic patients than in the general population. When it does occur in diabetic patients the underlying cause and its management are similar to that in non-diabetic patients.

Conclusions

Much has been learnt about the cause of hypertension in the diabetic individual in recent years. In IDDM patients, we now recognise that the development of hypertension is strongly linked to the development of nephropathy and that profound disturbances in blood pressure regulation are already apparent in the microalbuminuric phase of the disease. On the other hand, NIDDM patients account for the great majority of diabetic patients with hypertension and in these patients the cause of their hypertension is less clear cut. There is no doubt that obesity is the most important factor accounting for the high prevalence of hypertension in NIDDM, but it is not the sole explanation. Moreover, although the obesity-induced haemodynamic changes that result in hypertension appear to be well characterised, how obesity leads to these circulatory changes is still unresolved. Some have argued strongly that insulin resistance and the resulting hyperinsulinaemia is the causal link between obesity, glucose intolerance and hypertension. It is my own view that this concept is too simplistic and that, while some components of this hypothesis, e.g. sympathetic nervous system activation, may indeed be important, it is clear that there are other, as yet unidentified, pieces of this complex jigsaw.

REFERENCES

1. Nørgaard K, Feldt-Rasmussen B, Borch-Johnsen K, Sælan H, Deckert T. Prevalence of hypertension in type 1 (insulin-dependent) diabetes mellitus. *Diabetologia* 1990; **33**: 407-10.

2. Mathiesen ER, Rønn B, Jensen T, Storm B, Deckert T. Relationship between blood pressure and urinary albumin excretion in development of microalbuminuria. *Diabetes* 1990; **39**: 245-9.

3. Benhamou PY, Halimi S, De Gaudemaris R, Boizel R, Pitiot M, Siche JP, Bachelot I, Mallion JM. Early disturbances of ambulatory blood pressure load in normotensive type 1 diabetic patients with microalbuminuria. *Diabetes Care* 1992; **15** (11): 1614-9.

4. Christensen CK. Abnormal albuminuria and blood pressure rise in incipient diabetic nephropathy induced by exercise. *Kidney Int* 1984; **25**: 819-23.

5. Ferriss JB. The causes of raised blood pressure in insulin-dependent and non-insulin-dependent diabetes. *J Hum Hypertens* 1991; **5**: 245-54.

6. Feldt-Rasmussen B, Mathiesen ER, Deckert T, Giese J, Christensen NJ, Bent-Hansen L, Nielsen MD. Central role for sodium in the pathogenesis of blood pressure changes independent of angiotensin, aldosterone and catecholamines in type 1 (insulin-dependent) diabetes mellitus. *Diabetologia* 1987; **30**: 610-7.

7.   Poston L, Taylor PD. Endothelium-mediated vascular function in insulin-dependent diabetes mellitus. *Clin Sci* 1995; **88**: 245-55.

8. Goode GK, Miller JP, Heagerty AM. Hyperlipidaemia, hypertension, and coronary heart disease. *Lancet* 1995; **345**: 362-4.

9. Salomaa VV, Strandberg TE, Vanhanen H, Naukkarinen V, Sarna S, Miettinen TA. Glucose tolerance and blood pressure: long term follow up in middle aged men. *Br Med J* 1991; **302**: 493-6.

10. DeFronzo RA, Ferrannini E. Insulin resistance. A multifaceted syndrome responsible for NIDDM, obesity, hypertension, dyslipidaemia and atherosclerotic cardiovascular disease. *Diabetes Care* 1991; **14**: 173-94.

11. Williams B. Insulin resistance: the shape of things to come. *Lancet* 1994; **344**: 521-4.

12. Lindsay RS, Stewart MJ, Nairn IM, Baird JD, Padfield PL. Reduced diurnal variation of blood pressure in non-insulin-dependent diabetic patients with microalbuminuria. *J Hum Hypertens* 1995; **9**: 223-7.

13. Sawicki PT, Kaiser S, Heinemann L, Frenzel H, Berger M. Prevalence of renal artery stenosis in diabetes mellitus - an autopsy study. *J Int Med* 1991; **229**: 489-92.

CHAPTER TWO - SUMMARY POINTS

- The pathogenesis of hypertension differs in IDDM and NIDDM.
- Hypertension in IDDM is strongly related to the development of diabetic nephropathy.
- The development of persistent microalbuminuria signals a progressive rise in blood pressure in IDDM patients.
- Microalbuminuria is also associated with abnormal blood pressure regulation and a disturbed diurnal blood pressure variation.
- Hypertension is commonly present at diagnosis of NIDDM.
- Nephropathy is much less important as a primary cause of hypertension in NIDDM when compared to IDDM.
- Obesity is a major factor accounting for the hypertension of NIDDM, but other factors are also important.
- Exchangeable sodium is increased in both IDDM and NIDDM and is positively correlated with blood pressure.
- Glucose intolerance and hypertension are closely related variables.
- Always consider the possibility of secondary hypertension in diabetic patients.
- The prevalence of renal artery stenosis may be increased in NIDDM patients.

Chapter Three

DIABETES AND HYPERTENSION: A FATAL ATTRACTION

Introduction

Before the development of insulin therapy, most patients with insulin-dependent diabetes would have succumbed to the acute metabolic complications of the disease. With improvements in metabolic control, patients with diabetes mellitus have enjoyed a more prolonged life expectancy. It is now apparent, however, that a majority of diabetic patients will eventually die, often prematurely, due to the development of CV disease. An analysis of the complications that commonly occur in diabetic patients reveals that almost all of them can be attributed entirely, or predominantly, to accelerated vascular injury. Thus, although diabetes is classified as an endocrine disorder, the clinical consequences of diabetes are predominantly vascular. In this regard, diabetes mellitus can be regarded as a vascular disease and, as such, the complications of diabetes can be conveniently divided into macrovascular and microvascular complications (see Figure 6). The macrovascular complications are caused by the premature development of atherosclerosis resulting in ischaemia and thrombosis in a variety of vital organs. Diabetic microvascular disease is unique to this condition and is responsible for many of the devastating and debilitating complications of diabetes. In this chapter, I will first review the impact of diabetes mellitus on CV disease in general. Subsequently, I will describe how the interaction between diabetes and hypertension has been shown to increase, and in many cases greatly

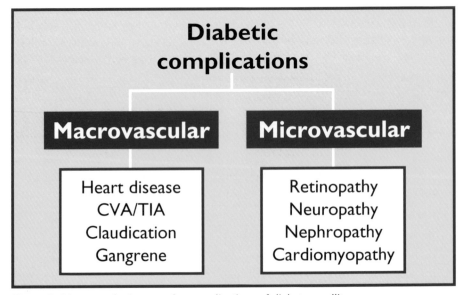

Figure 6 - Macro- and microvascular complications of diabetes mellitus.

accelerate, the development of the organ-specific manifestations of macrovascular and microvascular disease in patients with diabetes.

'Diabetes mellitus is a vascular disease'
It was over 40 years ago that Knud Lundbaek, while commenting on the fact that multiple diabetic complications often occurred together in the same patient, noted that:

> *'. . . the multiplicity of the interconnecting links between all the organ lesions (nephropathy, retinopathy and coronary disease), seems to indicate that the various anomalies are in reality various manifestations of one generalised vascular disease.'*

- K. Lundbaek, Lancet 1954.

The clinical presentation of the various complications of diabetes suggests that it is a disease of accelerated CV injury. This conclusion is borne out by the fact that CV disease and its consequences account for most of the excess and premature morbidity and mortality associated with both IDDM and NIDDM. The results of the Framingham study and other epidemiological studies have revealed the true potency of diabetes as a CV risk factor. From the Framingham data, the average annual age-adjusted incidence of CV disease was increased 2.2-fold in diabetic men and 2.8-fold in diabetic women when compared to the non-diabetic population (see Table 9)[1]. Similarly, CV disease mortality was massively increased in both diabetic men and women.

When the various categories of CV disease incidence are further analysed, it is apparent that the relative risk of a wide spectrum of CV events, including heart failure, CHD, CV disease and peripheral vascular disease, are all

Table 9 - The impact of diabetes mellitus on the average annual age-adjusted incidence/1,000 CV events in men and women aged 45-74 years from the Framingham cohort.

	Men		Women	
	Diabetic	Non-diabetic	Diabetic	Non-diabetic
CV disease	39.1	19.1	27.2	10.2
CV death	17.4	8.5	17.0	3.6
CHD	24.8	14.9	17.8	6.9
CCF	7.6	3.5	11.4	2.2
Claudication	12.6	3.3	8.4	1.3
CVA	4.7	1.9	6.2	1.7

Relative risks	Any CV disease		CV disease mortality		Cardiac failure		Brain infarct		Coronary disease		Intermittent claudication	
	M	F	M	F	M	F	M	F	M	F	M	F
Unadjusted	2.5	3.7	2.6	7.2	2.8	7.7	3.3	5.6	1.9	3.6	4.7	8.9
Age adjusted	2.2	2.8	2.1	4.9	2.2	5.4	2.7	3.8	1.7	2.7	4.0	6.4
Risk adjusted	2.1	2.0	1.7	3.3	1.8	3.8	2.2	2.2	1.7	2.1	4.2	5.0

markedly increased in diabetic patients (see Table 10)[1]. Even when the data are further adjusted for factors that may be represented in excess in the diabetic population (i.e. hypertension, hypercholesterolaemia, left ventricular hypertrophy and cigarette smoking), the relative risk for the entire spectrum of CV disease and CV death remains significantly elevated in the diabetic patients.

Thus, diabetes is a powerful, independent CV risk factor. One way of illustrating the potency of diabetes in this context is to compare diabetes with another recognised CV risk factor, e.g. cigarette smoking. This has been analysed from the Framingham database and the impact of diabetes on CV disease has been compared to smoking in a population of non-diabetic women. The results of this comparison, shown in Table 11[1], confirm that cigarette smoking (20 cigarettes per day) doubles the incidence of CV death and increases the incidence of the various individual categories of CV disease. However, when compared to diabetes, it is clear that diabetes is a much more potent CV risk factor than heavy cigarette smoking.

Hypertension is also a potent independent risk factor for CV disease and death. Hypertension is commonly associated with diabetes, particularly in NIDDM patients. This combination of hypertension with diabetes might reasonably be expected to increase a person's risk of developing CV disease. I will now review some of the evidence supporting the hypothesis that hypertension magnifies the already high CV risk associated with diabetes, thereby accelerating the development of both macrovascular and microvascular disease.

Table 11 - A comparison between the impact of diabetes and smoking on the average annual age-adjusted rate of specified events/1,000 at risk among women from the Framingham cohort. Diabetes is a more potent independent risk factor for cardiovascular disease than heavy smoking.

CV disease category	Diabetic non-smoker	Smoker (>20/day) non-diabetic	Non-smoker non-diabetic
CV disease	27.2	12.1	10.2
CV death	17.0	6.4	3.6
CHD	17.8	7.1	6.9
CCF	11.4	4.4	2.2
CVA	6.2	2.0	1.7
Claudication	8.4	2.9	1.3

Macrovascular disease

The development of atherosclerotic large-vessel disease or macrovascular disease is responsible for the high rates of CHD, CV disease and peripheral vascular disease in diabetic patients. Diabetes is a major independent risk factor for the development of macrovascular disease. Hypertension is also a potent risk factor for atherosclerosis and the combination of hypertension with diabetes greatly accelerates the pathogenesis of the life-threatening macrovascular complications of diabetes. The independent and combined contributions of diabetes and hypertension to the morbidity and mortality from CHD, CV disease and peripheral vascular disease are considered in more detail below.

Coronary heart disease (CHD)

Diabetes is a major independent risk factor for the development of CHD. Moreover, the diabetic patient is prone to a wide spectrum of clinical manifestations of CHD, including increased frequency of chronic silent ischaemia, acute silent or symptomatic myocardial infarction and acute complications of myocardial infarction. Diabetes also predisposes to increased short- and long-term mortality after acute infarction and increased rates of re-infarction and restenosis after angioplasty. The burden of diabetes with regard to CHD falls heavily on women in whom the presence of diabetes appears to nullify the 'cardiovascular protective' effect of the premenopausal years. Hypertension is also an important risk factor for CHD. A recent follow-up study examined the impact of SBP levels on CHD mortality over a 10-year period in almost 350,000 men which included over 5,000 with diabetes. CHD mortality was significantly higher in diabetic than non-diabetic patients at all values of blood pressure (see Figure 7)[2]. This demonstrates that hypertension accentuates the already high rate of CHD in diabetic patients and is supportive of previous studies which showed that the risk of CHD in diabetic patients is more than doubled by the co-existence of arterial hypertension.

Congestive cardiac failure (CCF)
In the Framingham cohort described above, the presence of diabetes was associated with a significantly greater incidence of CCF, the age-adjusted relative risk being 2.8 for men and 5.4 for women (Table 10). With longer follow-up, up to 30 years, these relative risk values had doubled. This implies that the disease process culminating in CCF is more severe in diabetic patients,

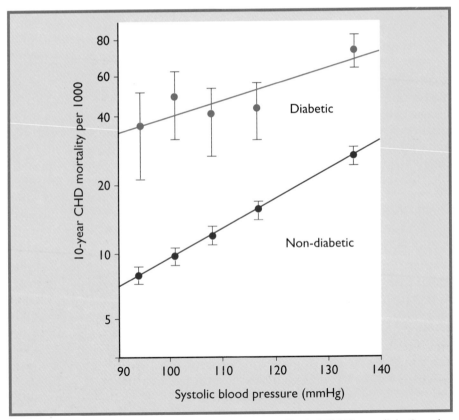

Figure 7 - Systolic blood pressure and 10-year CHD mortality in 342,815 non-diabetic and 5,163 diabetic men aged 35-57.

Diabetes and hypertension

perhaps indicating an 'accelerated ageing' of the hearts of diabetic patients. Consistent with this view, numerous non-invasive studies have revealed that diabetic patients have abnormalities in left ventricular function that are not attributable to coronary artery disease, indicating the possible existence of a specific diabetic cardiomyopathy.

Diabetic cardiomyopathy

The demonstration that diabetes predisposes to CCF has led to the proposal that a specific diabetes-induced cardiomyopathy exists. Impairment of both systolic and diastolic function have been described in diabetic patients with CCF and normal coronary arteries. Various histological abnormalities of the small intramural coronary vessels, with intimal proliferation and thickened walls, perivascular and interstitial fibrosis, and the accumulation of glycoproteins have all been reported as characteristic findings in diabetic cardiomyopathy. However, the changes described and the resulting myocardial fibrosis are pathologically similar to the fibrosis seen in hypertensive hearts and, clinically, diabetic cardiomyopathy is difficult to distinguish from hypertensive cardiomyopathy. Debate continues as to whether there is a specific diabetic cardiomyopathy or whether the aforementioned clinical and pathological features simply represent an exaggerated cardiac response to hypertension. It is my own view that the metabolic abnormalities of diabetes act in concert with elevated blood pressure to predispose to an accelerated development of myocardial hypertrophy and fibrosis, culminating in the premature onset of heart failure. Undoubtedly, the clinical severity of diabetic cardiomyopathy is greatly increased when hypertension and diabetes co-exist. Moreover, there is recent evidence to support the view that impaired glucose tolerance and hypertension interact to accelerate the development of left ventricular hypertrophy.

Left ventricular hypertrophy (LVH)

Left ventricular hypertrophy is ordinarily considered to be an important cardiac response to the sustained increases in peripheral vascular resistance observed in hypertensive patients. The development of LVH is an ominous sign as it is associated with a dramatically increased risk of CHD, sudden death (usually due to ventricular arrhythmias), CCF, stroke and peripheral vascular disease. When compared to hypertensive individuals without LVH, those with LVH are up to 10 times more likely to develop serious CV disease in general and CHD in particular. In this regard, LVH is seen as the most potent of all markers of coronary risk.

Several studies have suggested that diabetes may augment the development of LVH in hypertensive patients, some concluding that a high plasma glucose *per se* is an accelerating factor for LVH. More recently it has been shown that even at the preclinical stage of diabetes, i.e. glucose intolerance,

	Normotensive/ normal glucose tolerance	Hypertensive/ normal glucose tolerance	Hypertensive/ impaired glucose tolerance
Table 12 - Interaction between glucose intolerance and hypertension on the development of left ventricular hypertrophy (LVH). Hypertension significantly increases LVH (* = p<0.05) vs. normotensive subjects. The combination of glucose intolerance and hypertension significantly exaggerates the increase in LVH (+ = p<0.05 vs. hypertension and normal glucose tolerance).			
Left ventricular mass index (g/m²)	87.9±20.2	102.1±2.1*	115.6±28.2*+
Systolic BP (mmHg)	120±13	163±18	161±21*
Diastolic BP (mmHg)	69±10	93±11*	92±11*

the presence of glucose intolerance significantly increases the hypertrophic response of the left ventricle to essential hypertension (Table 12)[3].

The aforementioned data suggest that there is a potentially devastating interaction between the metabolic consequences of diabetes and the deleterious actions of hypertension on the structure and function of the heart. This interaction is apparent at the earliest indication of glucose intolerance and as a consequence of the mildest elevation of blood pressure. This may explain why such cardiac sequelae are so common in NIDDM patients, many of whom are hypertensive and have often experienced several years of glucose intolerance prior to the clinical diagnosis of NIDDM.

Cerebrovascular disease
Hypertension and diabetes are powerful independent risk factors for stroke and/or transient cerebral ischaemic episodes. The potency of diabetes as a major risk factor for the development of stroke was illustrated by the Framingham Heart Study, which demonstrated that after a 30-year follow-up of middle-aged men and women, diabetic men had 2.5 times the incidence of stroke compared to men without diabetes, and diabetic women had 3.6 times the incidence of stroke compared to the non-diabetic female population[4]. These conclusions have been substantiated by other large clinical trials and

epidemiological studies, all of which provide consistent data supporting the fact that the relative risk for stroke mortality and morbidity associated with diabetes is two to six times greater in both men and women compared to the non-diabetic population.

Hypertension is a major risk factor for stroke with a summary of recent trials suggesting that the presence of hypertension increases the risk of stroke by six times the average risk. Within a subset of patients who were both diabetic and hypertensive, stroke occurred twice as commonly as in those with hypertension alone. This confirms that the frequent co-existence of hypertension and diabetes leads to a substantial increase in the risk and prevalence of stroke.

Peripheral vascular disease

Autopsy studies and clinical anecdotes show that diabetic patients are more commonly and more severely affected by atherosclerosis in both the abdominal aorta and femoral arteries. This premature development of peripheral vascular disease usually manifests as intermittent claudication, but can result in rest pain, arterial foot ulceration, gangrene and infection, not infrequently culminating in lower limb amputation. A review of various studies suggests that a diabetic patient at the age of 70 years has a 70-fold increase in the risk of peripheral vascular disease when compared to a non-diabetic person of similar age. From prospective study data the relative risk of peripheral vascular disease in diabetic patients when compared to matched non-diabetic controls is increased up to three-fold in males and five- to eight-fold in females. The most important factors predicting the development of peripheral vascular disease in diabetics are:

- the duration of diabetes;
- a history of smoking;
- the presence of hypertension.

In older patients, there is indeed a very strong correlation between the prevalence of peripheral vascular disease and increased systolic blood pressure (SBP). It is unclear, however, whether the increase in SBP in these circumstances is causally related to the development of peripheral vascular disease or merely reflects the decreased compliance of diseased blood vessels. Nevertheless, there seems little doubt that the presence of hypertension greatly increases the risk of diabetic patients subsequently developing peripheral vascular disease.

Microvascular disease

Microvascular disease implies dysfunction and damage in capillary beds throughout the body. This injury to microvessels is often termed 'microangiopathy' and is characterised by the development of a widespread vascular injury that is unique to diabetes. Microvascular disease is most clinically apparent in the eye where it gives rise to a characteristic retinopathy. However, these pathological changes are not restricted to this site and are representative of a similar injurious process developing in microvascular beds elsewhere, such as the renal glomeruli (diabetic nephropathy), the vasovasorum of peripheral nervous tissue (diabetic neuropathy) and the myocardium (diabetic cardiomyopathy).

The pathogenesis of diabetic micro-angiopathy is incompletely understood and beyond the scope of this book. Nevertheless, haemodynamic and metabolic factors appear to be critically important in the initial pathogenesis of micro-angiopathy and its subsequent progression to overt disease. This implies that the excessive haemodynamic forces generated within the microcirculation as a consequence of hypertension could accelerate the development of micro-angiopathy in diabetic patients. A considerable body of evidence is now emerging to support this view.

Special vulnerability of the diabetic microcirculation to hypertensive injury
One of the characteristic pathological features of diabetes is the development of microvascular injury. This micro-angiopathy develops in the setting

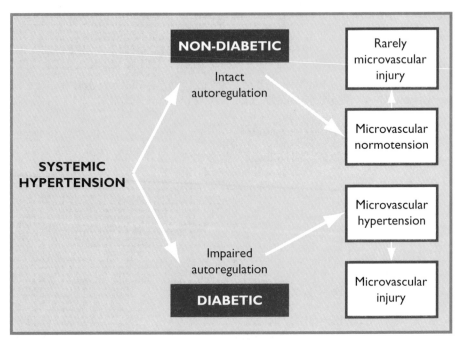

Figure 8 - Mechanism whereby impaired blood flow autoregulation leads to microvascular injury in diabetic patients.

Diabetes and hypertension

of seemingly normal systemic blood pressures and yet pathologically resembles injury that could have been produced as a consequence of microvascular hypertension. There is indeed a considerable body of evidence supporting the concept that microvascular pressures are abnormally high in diabetes and that microvascular hypertension may be the prime force leading to micro-angiopathy[5].

In the non-diabetic patient, hypertension does not usually promote the development of micro-angiopathy as the microcirculation is protected by blood flow autoregulation. This is an intrinsic reflex mechanism which causes the small afferent arterioles feeding the microcirculation to constrict when challenged by high perfusion pressures and thereby limits any pressure rise in the delicate capillary networks. Widespread abnormalities in blood flow autoregulation have now been demonstrated in many vascular beds in diabetic animals and people. This diabetes-induced abnormality in blood flow autoregulation means that for any given systemic blood pressure, microvascular pressures will be abnormally high. Thus, even mild elevations in blood pressure could potentially lead to marked increases in microvascular pressure. The loss of blood flow autoregulation in diabetic patients could thereby render the microcirculation of these subjects uniquely vulnerable to the development of hypertension (see Figure 8).

Support for this hypothesis comes from two intriguing clinical observations:

- The finding that the co-incidental development of renal artery stenosis in diabetic patients can protect against diabetic nephropathy in the kidney on the side of the stenosis, whereas nephropathy has developed in the contralateral kidney.

- Clinical reports of the unilateral development of diabetic retinopathy, the protected side being on the same side as a co-incidental carotid artery stenosis.

In both of these circumstances, the affected organs were all exposed to the metabolic consequences of diabetes, and injury developed unilaterally, only on the side exposed to normal systemic blood pressures. In effect, the fortuitous development of vascular stenosis provided crude blood flow autoregulation, limiting high perfusion pressures to the kidney and eye respectively and thereby protecting them from haemodynamic damage. These observations, subsequently verified by experimental studies, strongly support the hypothesis that haemodynamic forces are very important in the development of diabetic micro-angiopathy. Moreover, impaired autoregulation may explain why the microcirculation of diabetic patients is uniquely vulnerable to injury when hypertension co-exists.

Diabetic retinopathy

Diabetic retinopathy is a highly specific vascular complication of both IDDM and NIDDM, and is the most common cause of registered blindness in 35- to 65-year-old men and women in the UK and US. It has been estimated that 30-40,000 patients worldwide become blind each year as a consequence of diabetic retinopathy. The prevalence of diabetic retinopathy is strongly related to the duration of diabetes, suggesting that metabolic factors and in particular hyperglycaemia are important in its pathogenesis. However, the retina is also an important clinical barometer of target organ damage in hypertensive patients, and several anecdotal reports have long suggested an association between hypertension and the development of diabetic retinopathy. The best prospective study published to date examined the relationship between SBP and the incidence of diabetic retinopathy over six years in NIDDM patients. In this study, the incidence of retinal exudates was more than doubled in patients with a mean SBP of 145 mmHg or greater when compared to those

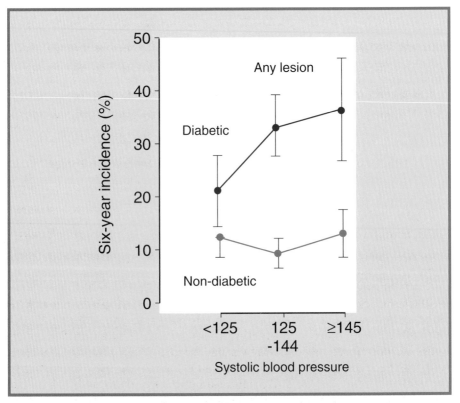

Figure 9 - Incidence of retinal exudates with increasing SBP (mmHg).

Diabetes and hypertension

	Glucose (mmol/l) (years)	Duration of diabetes	Systolic BP (mmHg)	Diastolic BP (mmHg)	Antihyper-tensive therapy
Retinopathy	8.8±0.4	10±0.8	172±5	93±2	44%
No retinopathy	8.9±0.3	18±0.7*	142±3*	80±2*	4%*

Table 13 - Risk factors for severe retinopathy in NIDDM patients. There are two groups: 50 patients with severe retinopathy (proliferative retinopathy or maculopathy) and 50 patients with no evidence of retinopathy. Differences in disease duration or metabolic control did not appear to account for the difference in severe retinopathy. The factor most strongly associated with retinopathy was the presence of hypertension (* = p<0.001).

whose SBP was less than 125 mmHg (see Figure 9)[6]. It is noteworthy that this dramatic increase in retinopathy was evident across a SBP range (i.e. 125-145 mmHg) that falls below the threshold SBP for antihypertensive therapy intervention in many currently published guidelines. In other studies examining the risk factors associated with the development of retinopathy in NIDDM patients, the coexistence of hypertension was the factor most strongly associated with the presence of severe diabetic retinopathy (see Table 13)[7].

In addition to classic retinopathy, diabetic patients are also prone to develop visual loss as a consequence of macular oedema, chronic open-angle glaucoma and ischaemic optic atrophy. Hypertension is an established risk factor for the development of macular oedema in patients with diabetes, probably because blood flow to the macular is substantially greater than that to the anterior retina. Thus, increased systemic blood pressure will increase retinal perfusion pressure, favouring the development of oedema in the highly perfused macular.

Chronic open-angle glaucoma is also more common in diabetic subjects. It has been suggested that diabetes-induced micro-angiopathy renders the optic nerve head more vulnerable to an elevation of the intra-ocular pressure which can produce optic nerve cupping, optic atrophy and visual field defects, thereby increasing the risk of blindness. Hypertension is a known risk factor for the development of ischaemic optic neuropathy. Thus, people with both diabetes and hypertension are at a higher risk for the development of both glaucoma and ischaemic optic neuropathy, than are diabetic patients who do not have hypertension.

The accumulating evidence suggests a powerful deleterious interaction between poor metabolic control and hypertension in the pathogenesis of the many manifestations of diabetic eye disease. Elevated blood pressure appears to be an important risk factor for the development of retinopathy, and this risk compounds the effect of poor metabolic control. In some small studies, controlling blood pressure appears to reduce the progression of diabetic retinopathy, but this awaits confirmation in larger prospective studies. It is indeed surprising that there have been few attempts to analyse the impact of hypertension and its treatment on this devastating consequence of diabetic micro-angiopathy.

Diabetic neuropathy

The pathogenesis of diabetic neuropathy is complex and more commonly develops in diabetic patients who:

- are male,

- have a history of poor metabolic control,

- have a long duration of their diabetes and

- are smokers.

The role of hypertension as a potential risk factor for the development of diabetic neuropathy remained obscure until the epidemiological correlations of diabetic neuropathy were more rigorously defined in a large study of IDDM patients from Pittsburgh, US (Figure 10)[8]. In patients with IDDM of 10-19 years duration, hypertension (>140/90 mmHg and/or taking antihypertensive medication), poor metabolic control and a low HDL-cholesterol concentration, were associated with a significantly greater prevalence of diabetic neuropathy. The presence of hypertension was associated with the highest prevalence of neuropathy and was detected in 28% of patients with neuropathy and only 10% without neuropathy. In IDDM patients of longer disease duration (≥20 years), smoking also became an important independent associate of increased prevalence of neuropathy. The demonstration that traditional CV risk factors, i.e. hypertension, smoking, dyslipidaemia and hyperglycaemia, are also associated with an increased prevalence of neuropathy, supports the concept that the pathogenesis of diabetic neuropathy, at least in part, relates to microvascular disease. It also raises the important question as to whether reducing the CV risk burden of patients with diabetes by treating hypertension and other risk factors may not only reduce overall CV morbidity and mortality, but also reduce the risk of diabetic neuropathy and its distressing clinical consequences.

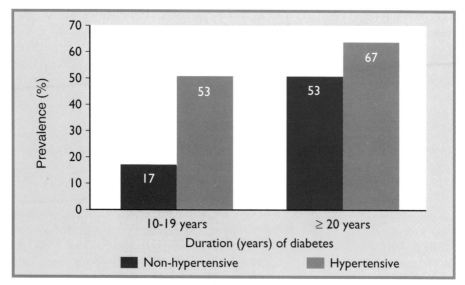

Figure 10 - Prevalence of neuropathy by duration of insulin-dependent diabetes. No neuropathy was detected at less than 10 years' duration.

Diabetic nephropathy

Diabetes mellitus is now the leading cause of end-stage renal disease in the Western world. The risk of diabetic renal disease increases with age and duration of diabetes. The development of nephropathy after 15 years of diabetes has been observed in more than 30% of IDDM patients and more than 20% of NIDDM patients. NIDDM patients represent by far the greater proportion of patients with diabetes, thus a majority of patients with diabetic nephropathy are in the NIDDM group. The subject of diabetic nephropathy will be considered in detail in Chapter 5. Nevertheless, it is worth emphasising at this point that diabetic nephropathy is a further example of how the development of microvascular disease can lead to devastating end-organ destruction, which ultimately impacts most unfavourably on patients' morbidity and mortality. It has long been recognised that the progression (i.e. deterioration in renal function) of many categories of renal disease is strongly influenced by the level of both systolic and diastolic blood pressure. It is not surprising, therefore, that the same is true for diabetic nephropathy. Moreover, hypertension is an early accompaniment of established proteinuria in patients with early evidence of diabetic nephropathy. The only prospective trials examining the impact of antihypertensive therapy on the progression of microvascular disease in diabetic patients have focused on diabetic nephropathy. This is because hypertension is common in patients with nephropathy, and also because changes in putative markers of renal injury and function, i.e. protein excretion and renal function, are relatively easy to document. Such studies have generated powerful evidence to suggest that prompt and effective treatment of hypertension in patients with evidence of diabetic nephropathy, even at its earliest stage (persistent microalbuminuria), can markedly delay the development of renal impairment (see Chapter 5).

Hypertension and mortality in diabetes mellitus

Cohort and insurance company data indicate that the mortality of diabetic patients increases with elevations of systolic and diastolic blood pressure. A seven-year mortality follow-up of almost 5,000 patients as part of the WHO Multinational Study of Vascular Disease in Diabetics (MSVDD) also showed that the level of blood pressure was independently related to circulatory disease mortality[9]. Over a seven-year follow-up, the risk of death was increased two-fold in hypertensive (BP ≥160/95 mmHg) IDDM and NIDDM patients. This effect on mortality was independent of the powerful influence of proteinuria on CV disease mortality. These findings were supported by the more recent London hypertension diabetes study group report in which hypertensive NIDDM patients showed a two-fold increase in diabetes-related death (predominantly CV events) compared with their age-matched normotensive counterparts[10]. Patients with hypertension and diabetes also had a 1.5-fold increased risk of developing a fatal or non-fatal morbid event. This association between hypertension and death was statistically significant independent of other risk factors, such as smoking, age, gender and lipid abnormalities, with a hazard ratio of 1.9 for death. These studies strongly suggest that hypertension increases the mortality of patients with diabetes.

Diabetes and hypertension, a 'fatal attraction'

As indicated above, both diabetes and hypertension have the capacity to influence CV risk adversely. The aforementioned evidence suggests a pathogenic mechanism whereby the metabolic consequences of diabetes act to increase the vulnerability of the vasculature to injury, thereby 'setting the stage' for hypertension to accelerate that injurious process. This is classically illustrated by the capacity of metabolic factors to impair blood flow autoregulation, and thus render the microcirculation of diabetic patients especially vulnerable to systemic hypertension. This scenario may also help to explain why even mild elevations of blood pressure seemingly produce such devastating effects in diabetic patients. Thus, hypertension and diabetes, two of nature's most powerful CV risk factors, are inextricably linked, potentiate each other's adverse effects and thereby form the basis of a 'fatal attraction' that accounts for the vast majority of the morbidity and mortality experienced by patients with diabetes.

REFERENCES

1. Kannel WB, McGee DL. Diabetes and glucose tolerance as risk factors for cardiovascular disease: the Framingham Study. *Diabetes Care* 1979; **2**: 120-6.

2. Stamler J, Vaccaro O, Neaton JD, Wentworth D. Diabetes, other risk factors and 12-year cardiovascular mortality for men screened in the multiple risk factor intervention trial. *Diabetes Care* 1993; **16** :434-44.

3. Hara-Nakamura N, Kohara K, Sumimoto T, Lin M, Hiwada K. Glucose intolerance exaggerates left ventricular hypertrophy and dysfunction in essential hypertension. *Am J Hypertens* 1994; **7**: 1110-4.

4. Wolf PA, Kannel WB. Reduction of stroke through risk factor modification. *Semin Neurol* 1986; **6**: 243-53.

5. Tooke JE. Microvascular haemodynamics in diabetes mellitus. *Clin Sci* 1986; **70**: 119-25.

6. Knowler WC, Bennett PH, Ballintine EJ. Increased incidence of retinopathy in diabetics with elevated blood pressure: a six year follow-up study in Pima Indians. *N Engl J Med* 1980; **302**: 645-50.

7. Barnett AH, Britton JR, Leatherdale BA. Study of possible risk factors for severe retinopathy in non-insulin dependent diabetes. *Br Med J* 1983; **287**: 529.

8. Maser RE, Steenkiste AR, Dorman JS, Nielsen VK, Bass EB, Manjoo Q, Drash AL, Becker DJ, Kuller LH, Greene DA, Orchard TJ. Epidemiological correlates of diabetic neuropathy. Report from Pittsburgh Epidemiology of Diabetes Complications Study. *Diabetes* 1989; **38**: 1456-61.

9. Fuller JH, Head J, WHO Multinational Study Group. Blood pressure, proteinuria and their relationship with circulatory mortality: the WHO multinational study of vascular disease in diabetics. *Diabete Metab* 1989; **15**: 273-7.

10. The Hypertension in Diabetes Study Group. Hypertension in Diabetes Study (HDS): II. Increased risk of cardiovascular complications in hypertensive type 2 diabetic patients. *J Hypertens* 1993; **11**: 319-25.

CHAPTER 3 - SUMMARY POINTS

- Diabetes mellitus can be considered a 'vascular disease'.
- The major complications of diabetes are due to vascular disease.
- Macrovascular complications include CHD, cerebrovascular disease and peripheral vascular disease.
- Microvascular complications include retinopathy, nephropathy, neuropathy and cardiomyopathy.
- The duration of diabetes and degree of metabolic control have a major impact on the prevalence and progression of micro- and macrovascular disease.
- Hypertension is common in diabetic patients.
- Hypertension appears to act synergistically to accelerate the development of vascular disease in diabetic patients.
- The diabetic microcirculation may be especially vulnerable to systemic hypertension because of impaired blood flow autoregulation.
- Cardiovascular disease is the major cause of morbidity and death in patients with diabetes.

Chapter Four

DIABETES MELLITUS: A CONSPIRACY OF CARDIOVASCULAR RISK FACTORS

Introduction

The risk of a hypertensive patient suffering a cardiovascular (CV) event is not only related to the level of blood pressure, but also to the presence of associated risk factors for CV disease. Many CV risk factors have been identified (see Figure 11), and it is inevitable that most patients with diabetes will possess at least one (i.e. hyperglycaemia) and probably others (i.e. dyslipidaemia, obesity and left ventricular hypertrophy [LVH]) which will greatly magnify the risk of a CV event at any given level of blood pressure (Figure 12 - the 'Framingham graph'). The metabolic basis of NIDDM is insulin resistance, and it has been proposed that insulin resistance and the resulting hyperinsulinaemia may be responsible for the clustering of CV risk factors that ultimately predisposes to the high CV morbidity and mortality experienced by these patients.

What is insulin resistance?

Insulin resistance is defined as impaired sensitivity to the actions of insulin on whole body glucose utilisation. The precise characterisation of insulin sensitivity requires the use of the euglycaemic clamp, but in large epidemiological studies it is often inferred from the measurement of fasting plasma glucose and insulin concentrations. In such circumstances, an inappropriately high plasma insulin:glucose ratio is indicative of insulin resistance. Numerous studies have confirmed that there is tremendous variability in insulin sensitivity within seemingly normal healthy populations. At any given age, insulin sensitivity may vary by as much as seven-fold and insulin sensitivity diminishes with age (see Figure 13)[1]. This means that as many as 25% of the non-diabetic population have the same level of insulin resistance as people with impaired glucose tolerance or NIDDM. The only difference is that the non-diabetic individuals are able to compensate for their insulin

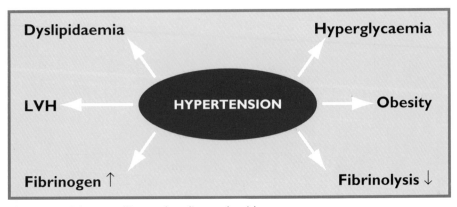

Figure 11 - Diabetes mellitus and cardiovascular risk.

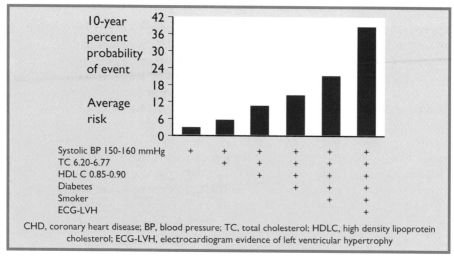

10-year percent probability of event						
Systolic BP 150-160 mmHg	+	+	+	+	+	+
TC 6.20-6.77		+	+	+	+	+
HDL C 0.85-0.90			+	+	+	+
Diabetes				+	+	+
Smoker					+	+
ECG-LVH						+

CHD, coronary heart disease; BP, blood pressure; TC, total cholesterol; HDLC, high density lipoprotein cholesterol; ECG-LVH, electrocardiogram evidence of left ventricular hypertrophy

Figure 12 - Probability of CHD event in mild hypertension by associated risk factors (men aged 45 years). Based on data from Framingham Study.

resistance by adequately increasing their insulin secretion. Thus, normal glucose tolerance is maintained in these individuals at the expense of hyperinsulinaemia. It is only when the compensatory increase in insulin secretion becomes inadequate that glucose intolerance, and subsequently NIDDM, develop. This means that the metabolic abnormality of insulin

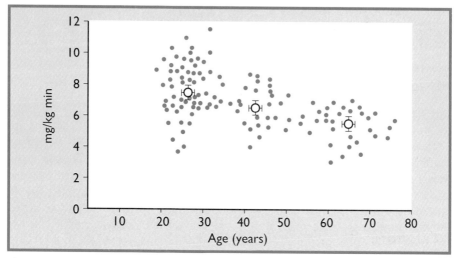

Figure 13 - Insulin mediated glucose disposal in healthy subjects.

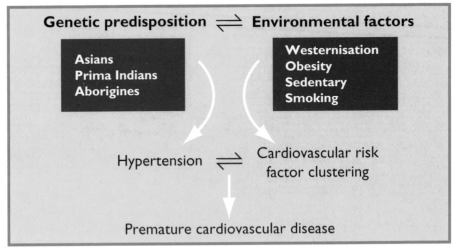

Figure 14 -The basis of insulin resistance.

resistance and hyperinsulinaemia often precedes the diagnosis of NIDDM by many years. It also means that the clustering of CV risk factors associated with insulin resistance, including hypertension, antedates the development of NIDDM. This perhaps explains why so many patients already have hypertension and established vascular disease when NIDDM is first diagnosed.

The basis of insulin resistance

Insulin resistance may be genetically determined and/or acquired (see Figure 14). The genetic basis may in part account for the high prevalence of insulin resistance and consequent NIDDM in certain racial groups, e.g. 'Westernised' Asian people. The precise mode of inheritance and the cellular basis of the defect are still unclear.

Insulin resistance is most commonly acquired as the result of obesity, a sedentary lifestyle and ageing. Insulin-mediated glucose disposal declines by 30-40% when an individual is 40% over ideal body weight. Indeed body fat, and in particular its distribution, are very powerful determinants of an individual's insulin sensitivity. In my opinion, reference to body mass index (BMI) alone as an index of obesity is inadequate because the distribution of body fat as well as the absolute amount of fat has a crucial impact on its metabolic consequences. Upper body obesity or central obesity is linked to the accumulation of visceral fat. It is visceral fat accumulation that is most strongly linked to insulin resistance. Indeed, the use of computerised tomography (CT) scanning to quantify visceral fat accurately has demonstrated remarkably tight correlations between visceral fat levels and insulin

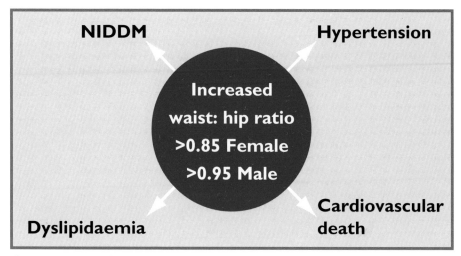

Figure 15 - Increased waist/hip ratio and its associated risks.

sensitivity. This is true even when young, lean and healthy individuals are examined. Anthropometric measurements such as the waist:hip ratio (WHR) are a useful surrogate for central obesity and thus a better clinical predictor of insulin resistance and CV risk-factor clustering than BMI measurements. As body fat distribution strongly predicts insulin sensitivity, it also predicts an individual's likelihood of acquiring a clustering of undesirable CV risk factors. This probably explains the strong association between central adiposity and CV morbidity and mortality. Figure 15 shows that the presence of increased central obesity, as indicated by an increased WHR, is strongly predictive of the likelihood of developing hypertension, glucose intolerance, NIDDM and dyslipidaemia, and of suffering a CV death.

Cardiovascular risk-factor clustering associated with diabetes mellitus: the role of insulin resistance

Diabetes and dyslipidaemia

When discussing diabetes, the term dyslipidaemia is preferred to hyperlipidaemia because some of the important lipid changes in diabetes relate to a reduction in the level of a specific lipid moiety, i.e. HDL-cholesterol.

Specific lipid abnormalities are uncommon or absent in IDDM patients with good glycaemic control. Triglycerides may be increased, but usually fall on treatment with insulin because of an insulin-stimulated increase in lipoprotein lipase activity.

NIDDM patients most commonly develop lipid abnormalities. In these patients high triglycerides are frequently noted, often in combination with

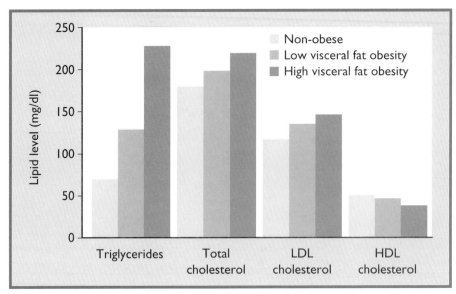

Figure 16 - Relationship between visceral obesity and dyslipidaemia.

a low HDL-cholesterol. This pattern of dyslipidaemia has been strongly related to CHD risk. Hypertriglyceridaemia may be directly atherogenic and HDL-cholesterol is recognised to be protective against vascular disease; thus low HDL-levels are an undesirable development. In non-diabetic and diabetic individuals there is considerable evidence supporting the hypothesis that insulin resistance and/or hyperinsulinaemia plays an important role in the development of this pattern of dyslipidaemia. If this is true, then one would expect to see a strong correlation between visceral obesity and lipid levels because visceral obesity is a powerful determinant of insulin sensitivity. Figure 16 shows that increasing levels of visceral obesity are indeed associated with higher triglyceride and lower HDL-cholesterol levels. Insulin resistance is also common in non-diabetic hypertensive subjects, even without co-existent overt obesity. The same pattern of dyslipidaemia is also observed in these individuals, supporting the concept that these lipid changes are in some way driven by insulin resistance and/or hyperinsulinaemia.

The distribution of plasma cholesterol and LDL concentrations in diabetic populations (IDDM and NIDDM) is similar to that in the general population. However, there are important qualitative changes in the LDL of diabetic patients that may render the LDL more atherogenic. In diabetes, the LDL is modified by oxidation and glycosylation and the LDL particles of diabetic patients are smaller and more dense. Each of these changes can lead to

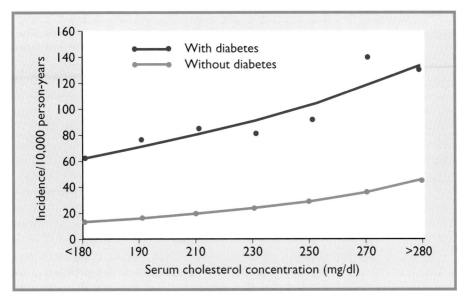

Figure 17 - Incidence of coronary mortality in relation to plasma cholesterol observed in men with or without diabetes in the Multiple Risk-Factor Intervention Trial (MRFIT). Based on data from MRFIT.

increased atherogenicity of the LDL particle. This may explain why in the Multiple Risk-Factor Intervention Trial (MRFIT), the incidence of CHD mortality was four-fold greater at any given cholesterol level when compared to the non-diabetic population (see Figure 17)[2].

Abnormalities in blood clotting and clot lysis

Fibrinolysis: The formation of a blood clot within a diseased vessel is often a final event in vascular occlusion, i.e. a coronary vessel occlusion leading to myocardial infarction. There is considerable evidence to suggest that insulin resistance and perhaps the resulting hyperinsulinaemia may play a key role in generating a pro-coagulant state on the endothelial surface. Under normal conditions, clot formation and lysis is finely regulated. Lysis is achieved by activation of the fibrinolytic pathway. This fibrinolytic system is naturally inhibited by plasminogen activator inhibitor-1 (PAI-1). In insulin-resistant states, including NIDDM, PAI-1 levels are elevated thereby generating a hypofibrinolytic state. This subtle change means that any clots forming within the circulation are less likely to be lysed and therefore more likely to promote vascular occlusion.

Platelet function: Platelets are crucial to thrombus formation and have also been implicated in the early stage of atheroma formation via the release of growth factors such as platelet-derived growth factor (PDGF).

Risk factor conspiracy

Various reports have suggested that platelet adhesion and aggregation are increased in both IDDM and NIDDM patients. These latter changes have not been linked to insulin resistance *per se* and they most likely represent modifications in platelet structure and function related to other abnormalities in diabetes, such as hyperglycaemia or dyslipidaemia. It is of interest that platelet function seems to be most notably disturbed in diabetic patients with microalbuminuria or proteinuria.

Fibrinogen: Fibrinogen is a soluble clotting factor, the blood level of which has been strongly and positively correlated with the risk of suffering a myocardial infarction. IDDM and NIDDM patients are more likely to have increased fibrinogen levels when compared to the non-diabetic population. The mechanism for this change is unknown, but the level of fibrinogen is directly correlated with glycaemia. Thus hyperglycaemia is associated with a higher fibrinogen level. Fibrinogen levels are also elevated by approximately 25% in diabetic patients with nephropathy (proteinuria) and, to a lesser degree, in patients with incipient nephropathy or microalbuminuria.

Von Willebrand factor (factor VIII): Von Willebrand factor is a glycoprotein synthesised by endothelial cells, and high circulating levels represent endothelial injury. When released from the endothelium it promotes the adhesion of platelets to the sub-endothelium. Circulating Von Willebrand factor levels are increased in IDDM and NIDDM patients. The circulating level of this factor is not influenced by glycaemic control and it appears to be a subtle early marker of endothelial injury as it is usually elevated in those patients with clinical evidence of microvascular injury, microalbuminuria and proteinuria.

Lipoprotein (a) (Lp[a]): Lp(a) should also be mentioned in relation to blood clotting. Lp(a) resembles LDL but also has a plasminogen-like molecule within its structure. It has been suggested that, when circulating levels of Lp(a) are increased, it could compete with plasminogen and thereby reduce fibrinolysis. Such a mechanism may explain why high Lp(a) levels have been associated with an increased risk of atherosclerosis. There are conflicting data in the literature as to whether Lp(a) levels are specifically increased in diabetic subjects. My assessment of this literature is that Lp(a) levels are not increased by diabetes *per se*, but they are increased in diabetic patients with microalbuminuria or overt renal disease (proteinuria).

The aforementioned data suggest that diabetes is associated with multiple abnormalities in the blood clotting and clot lysis cascades. Some of these abnormalities appear to be related to insulin resistance and hyperglycaemia, i.e. increased PAI-1 levels and increased fibrinogen. Others are more generally related to diabetes, i.e. increased platelet adhesion and aggregation, and increased Von Willebrand factor release. Some of the changes are particularly pronounced in diabetic patients with microalbuminuria or proteinuria,

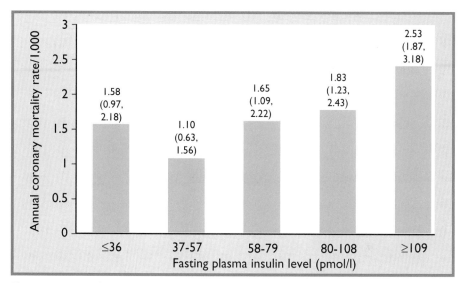

Figure 18 - Annual coronary mortality rates over 15 years of follow-up in relation to fasting plasma insulin quintiles measured at entry into the Paris prospective study. The actual mortality rate/1,000 and the confidence intervals (in parentheses) are given as numbers above each bar.

i.e. platelet functional changes, Von Willebrand factor release and increased Lp(a), which may contribute to the massive excess of CV disease in patients with nephropathy (see Chapter 5).

A possible direct atherogenic effect of insulin?
Insulin resistance precedes the diagnosis of NIDDM, often by many years. During this time the 'pre-diabetic' individual will be chronically exposed to abnormally high insulin levels in an endeavour to overcome the insulin resistance and maintain normal glucose tolerance. At least three prospective epidemiological studies have shown that hyperinsulinaemia is associated with atherosclerosis in the general population (Figures 18[3] and 19[4]). This kind of observation has led some to suggest that insulin may itself be pro-atherogenic and promote the development of vascular disease. I would dispute this view and suggest that insulin levels are a marker for insulin resistance and that the CV risk-factor clustering associated with insulin resistance accounts for the excess CV disease, rather than any direct effect of insulin on the atheromatous disease process.

Hyperglycaemia and atherosclerosis
Elevated blood glucose levels are in direct contact with vascular structures in diabetic subjects. Multiple biochemical pathways have been identified whereby glucose could modify various biological functions within vascular

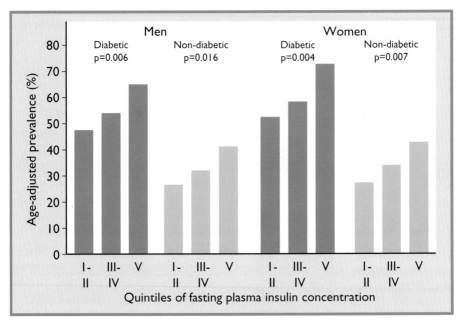

Figure 19 - Prevalence of clinical coronary artery disease and/or ischaemic ECG changes in men and women in relation to their fasting insulin quintiles. The association of coronary artery disease with increasing insulin levels exists in both sexes and in those with and without diabetes.

cells. Moreover, glycosylation and the formation of advanced glycosylation end products can also alter the structure of various molecules within the vessels' wall and unfavourably influence vascular function. Data from the Framingham study have already established hyperglycaemia as an independent CV risk factor. In this context, it seems likely that glucose is not only functioning as a marker of insulin resistance and the attendant CV risk factors, but also as a direct vascular toxin.

Insulin resistance and cardiovascular risk-factor clustering
It is beginning to look as though many, but not all, of the CV risk factors associated with NIDDM, develop in association with insulin resistance (see Figure 20). Thus, the clock is ticking and a cocktail of inter-related CV risk factors is assembled long before NIDDM is recognised or diagnosed in the patient. This prolonged period of insulin resistance is often clinically silent and has been termed 'the silent killer'. The pathological significance of this 'silent' period has been dramatically illustrated by the study of Asian migrants living in the United Kingdom, in whom insulin resistance develops via the combined effects of genetic predisposition and the adverse environmental influences of rapid 'Westernisation'.

Risk factor conspiracy

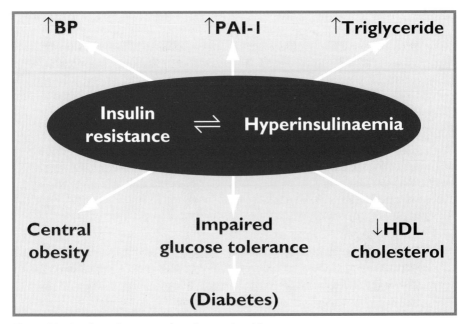

Figure 20 - Insulin resistance and cardiovascular risk.

Insulin resistance and cardiovascular disease in 'Westernised' Asian communities

Migrant Asian people living in the UK have a much higher prevalence of NIDDM (20% of the Asian community in some areas) than the indigenous population (<5%), and much higher rates of death from ischaemic heart disease and stroke[5,6]. Moreover, while CHD death rates have been falling over the past two decades in most of the western world, they have continued rising in 'Westernised' Asian people. In these communities, markers of recently acquired central adiposity and decreased levels of physical activity are prominent. Not surprisingly, therefore, insulin resistance and the associated risk-factor clustering are also very common. Various studies have shown a strong association between the development of insulin resistance and increased blood levels of triglyceride, and decreased levels of HDL-cholesterol in the western Asian communities. It is also important to note that the BMI of the Asian communities was often found to be lower than the BMI of the indigenous European population, but the waist:hip ratio measurements were greater in Asian people. This illustrates the insensitivity of the BMI measurement to detect central adiposity and the fact that anthropometric measurements which more accurately determine the distribution of body fat are more strongly predictive of insulin resistance, CV risk and the likely development of

NIDDM. There is another point of interest from these studies of Asian communities in the West. It is notable that their increased CV morbidity and mortality often occurs despite blood pressure levels which are not consistently higher, and are often lower, than those of the indigenous population. This observation illustrates the powerful independent effects of the adverse CV risk-factor profile associated with diabetes and the potential for it to be further magnified by the development of hypertension.

'Diabetes mellitus is a conspiracy of cardiovascular risk factors'

The aforementioned information illustrates that diabetic patients acquire an unenviable list of CV risk factors that greatly increase their overall risk of developing CV disease. Add to this the high prevalence of hypertension and it is easy to appreciate why CV disease is so common in these patients. Four further points are important with regard to the impact of hypertension:

1. Although many of the aforementioned changes appear subtle, their chronicity greatly increases their potency. It is noteworthy that many of these changes will have been present long before the diagnosis of NIDDM, and their CV impact cannot be overstated.

2. The CV risk factors do not occur in isolation; on the contrary, they tend to cluster and this clustering greatly magnifies their potency. Figure 11 illustrates how the adverse effects of hypertension are greatly magnified by the clustering of risk factors associated with diabetes. CV risk in hypertensive patients is concentrated on those with associated risk factors.

3. The fact that hypertension is associated with such a conspiracy of risk factors in the diabetic patient emphasises the need to address and attempt to modify as many of these risk factors as possible when managing these patients. It is only this whole patient approach that is likely to succeed in reducing the burden of risk.

4. Finally, certain classes of antihypertensive medication, most notably higher-dose thiazide diuretics and beta-blockers, have the potential to exacerbate the insulin resistance syndrome and thus accentuate the associated CV risk-factor clustering. The CV significance of this effect is unclear. However, some have suggested that these adverse metabolic effects could account for the shortfall in the reduction of myocardial infarction in the large, prospective antihypertensive therapy trials that have used higher-dose thiazide diuretics and beta-blockers. In this regard, the newer classes of antihypertensive therapy do not induce

insulin resistance and remain metabolically neutral - calcium channel blockers, ACE inhibitors and alpha₁-adrenoceptor antagonists may actually improve insulin sensitivity. Whether the more favourable metabolic effects of these newer agents translates into greater efficacy in reducing CV events awaits confirmation.

REFERENCES

1. DeFronzo RA, Ferrannini E. Insulin resistance. A multifaceted syndrome responsible for NIDDM, obesity, hypertension, dyslipidaemia and atherosclerotic cardiovascular disease. *Diabetes Care* 1991; **14**: 173-94.

2. Stamler J, Vaccaro O, Neaton JD, Wentworth D. Diabetes, other risk factors and 12 year cardiovascular mortality for men screened in the Multiple Risk Factor Intervention Trial. *Diabetes Care* 1993; **16**: 434-44.

3. Fontbonne A, Charles MA, Thibult N et al. Hyperinsulinaemia as a predictor of coronary heart disease mortality in a healthy population: the Paris prospective study, 15 year follow-up. *Diabetologia* 1991; **34**: 356-61.

4. Rönnemaa T, Laakso M, Pyörälä K *et al*. High fasting plasma insulin is an indicator of coronary heart disease in non-insulin-dependent diabetic patients and non-diabetic subjects. *Arterioscler Thromb* 1991; **11**: 80-90.

5. Williams B. Insulin resistance: the shape of things to come. *Lancet* 1994; **344**: 521-4.

6. Williams B. Westernised Asians and cardiovascular disease: nature or nurture? *Lancet* 1995; **345**: 401-2.

CHAPTER 4 - SUMMARY POINTS

- Cardiovascular risk is concentrated on hypertensive patients with multiple risk factors.
- Most people with diabetes have multiple risk factors for cardiovascular disease (e.g. hyperglycaemia, dyslipidaemia, obesity and left ventricular hypertrophy).
- Insulin resistance is associated with cardiovascular risk factor clustering.
- Insulin resistance is genetically determined and/or acquired due to the development of central obesity.
- Waist:hip ratio measurements are a more accurate determinant of insulin resistance than BMI.
- The dyslipidaemia of insulin resistance is characterised by hypertriglyceridaemia and low HDL-cholesterol levels.
- 'Westernised' Indo-Asians exhibit the features of insulin resistance and are prone to premature cardiovascular disease.
- Successful management of hypertension involves the management of all cardiovascular risk factors.
- Non-pharmacological strategies (e.g. weight reduction, increased physical exercise) are important in the management of patients with diabetes.
- The pharmacological management of hypertension in individuals with diabetes should avoid agents that potentially exacerbate the insulin resistance syndrome, particularly in those so predisposed.

Risk factor conspiracy

Chapter Five

DIABETIC NEPHROPATHY, MICROALBUMINURIA AND PROTEINURIA

Introduction

Diabetic nephropathy plays a very significant role in the development of hypertension and is an important cause of morbidity and mortality, particularly in IDDM, but also in NIDDM patients. Diabetic nephropathy is associated with an increase in urinary protein excretion. It is important to appreciate that this increase in urinary excretion of protein not only heralds the onset of diabetic nephropathy, but also potently predicts the premature death of diabetic patients from cardiovascular (CV) disease. In other words, microalbuminuria and proteinuria are not just markers of renal disease; they are also strong predictors of the likelihood that the diabetic individual will be hypertensive and will die prematurely from CV disease.

This chapter will provide an overview of diabetic nephropathy in clinical practice, and will then discuss the wider implications of microalbuminuria and proteinuria with regard to hypertension and CV disease.

Definition and epidemiology of diabetic nephropathy

Diabetic nephropathy occurs in both IDDM and NIDDM patients, and results in characteristic physiological and pathological changes within the kidney. Typical morphological changes of advanced diabetic nephropathy are similar in IDDM and NIDDM, and include:

- Basement membrane thickening.

- Mesangial matrix expansion (leading to diffuse glomerulosclerosis).

- Characteristic 'nodular' sclerotic lesion (the Kimmelstein-Wilson lesion).

The diagnosis is only definitively made by renal biopsy, but this is rarely necessary in clinical practice where the diagnosis is based on the recognition of the 'clinical triad' of diabetic nephropathy, i.e.:

- the presence of proteinuria,

- the development of a progressive rise in blood pressure, and

- a progressive and relentless decline in renal function towards end-stage renal failure (see Figure 21).

In a majority of patients, microvascular disease and macrovascular disease are well established in other tissues when diabetic nephropathy becomes clinically apparent. This means that diabetic retinopathy is invariably present. This had led to the suggestion that if diabetic retinopathy is not present in a patient with the diagnostic triad of diabetic nephropathy, then an alternative explanation for the renal disease is likely.

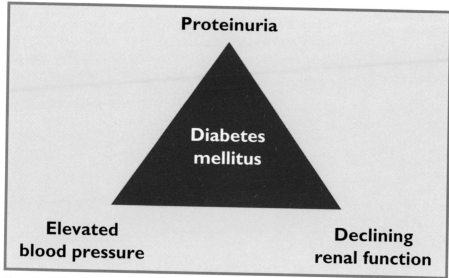

Figure 21 - The 'clinical triad' of diabetic nephropathy.

Clinical diabetic nephropathy occurs most commonly in IDDM; nevertheless, because the ratio of NIDDM to IDDM patients approximates to 10:1, most patients with chronic renal impairment due to diabetic nephropathy have NIDDM rather than IDDM. The clinical syndrome and epidemiology of diabetic nephropathy have been most extensively studied in IDDM patients. As an increase in protein excretion is the hallmark of diabetic nephropathy, the clinical diagnosis has traditionally been based on the presence of proteinuria on a standard bedside urine dipstick test. However, with more sensitive methods for assaying urine protein excretion rates, increases in protein excretion can be detected much earlier (see microalbuminuria). The increased urinary albumin excretion rate of patients with microalbuminuria eventually progresses with time to proteinuria. Thus, the terminology for diabetic nephropathy reflects this with the introduction of the label 'incipient nephropathy' for those with microalbuminuria and 'nephropathy' for those with proteinuria. This terminology has been useful for characterising the different clinical phases of diabetic nephropathy. Figure 22 illustrates a simplified view of the natural history of diabetic nephropathy.

Microalbuminuria will develop in some, but not all, IDDM patients, usually after a latent period of at least five years from diagnosis. Microalbuminuria will be present in approximately 5-10% of NIDDM patients at the time of diagnosis. At this early micro-albuminuric stage in IDDM and NIDDM, renal function, as determined by measurement of serum creatinine, will appear normal but the early pathological changes of diabetic nephropathy are already developing

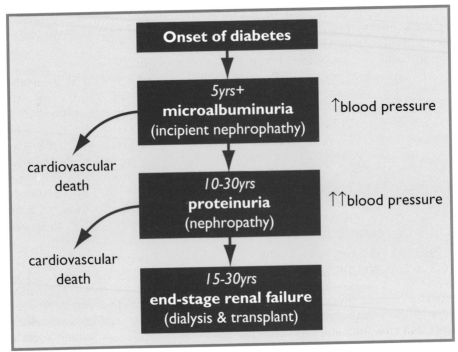

Figure 22 - Natural history of diabetic nephropathy.

within the renal glomeruli. The glomerular filtration rate (GFR) is usually normal at this stage and may be high due to hyperfiltration, but it is soon destined to begin a relentless decline. It is also at this stage that abnormalities in blood pressure regulation are becoming apparent (see Table 5) and that blood pressure begins a progressive and relentless rise, paralleling the rise in albumin excretion. The blood pressure level may, however, remain within the arbitrarily defined 'normal' range for a number of years.

After a further time lapse of five to 10 years, during which there is a year-on-year rise in albumin excretion (averaging 20% per year), a significant number of patients with microalbuminuria are eventually identified as having proteinuria. At this stage, a vast majority of patients will be overtly hypertensive and their renal function, as assessed by serum creatinine, may already be abnormal. (Serum creatinine is a very insensitive marker of renal functional impairment. A significant amount [probably >50% of functional renal tissue] has to be lost before an increment in serum creatinine becomes apparent.) When proteinuria is established, the patient's renal function will begin an inexorable decline towards end-stage renal failure, dialysis, transplantation or death.

Diabetic nephropathy

The pathogenesis of diabetic nephropathy has been best characterised for IDDM, but recent studies in NIDDM patients suggest that microalbuminuria is similarly predictive of nephropathy and that the pathogenesis of nephropathy is little different from that described for IDDM.

The rate of decline of GFR, once nephropathy (proteinuria) is established, does appear to differ between IDDM and NIDDM. In IDDM it approximates to a loss of GFR of 10 ml/min/year; thus, assuming a baseline GFR of 100-120 ml/min, IDDM patients will usually be on dialysis within 10 years of the onset of proteinuria, providing they do not succumb to CV disease along the way. NIDDM patients with proteinuria have been estimated to lose their GFR at 5-6 ml/min/year. However, GFR declines naturally with age, so the older NIDDM patients have a lower baseline GFR and usually reach end-stage renal failure within 10 years of the onset of proteinuria. Thus, if IDDM or NIDDM patients are destined to develop overt nephropathy, they will usually do so within 10-20 years of their diagnosis.

In recent years, it has become apparent that the development of microalbuminuria and proteinuria is not only indicative of nephropathy but is also strongly predictive of a premature death from CV disease, usually myocardial infarction, particularly in NIDDM patients. Thus, proteinuria in NIDDM patients tends to predict a premature death from CV disease before sufficient time has elapsed for nephropathy to develop. Moreover, even if diabetic patients with nephropathy survive until end-stage renal failure develops, and commence dialysis or receive a renal transplant, their prognosis is considerably worse than that of non-diabetic subjects on renal replacement therapy. This poor prognosis reflects the gross excess of CV disease in diabetic patients with nephropathy. Thus, for diabetic patients on the slippery slope of nephropathy, the outlook is bleak unless they are identified early and the management of their clinical condition is optimised. In this latter regard, the appropriate management of patients' hypertension appears to be crucial (see Chapters 6 and 7).

How many diabetic subjects get diabetic nephropathy?
Fortunately, not all patients with diabetes get nephropathy. In IDDM patients, the cumulative incidence of nephropathy is usually quoted to be 35-40%; thus approximately one-third of IDDM patients are ultimately affected. More recent data suggest that there may be a declining incidence of nephropathy in IDDM patients, with only 25% of patients developing nephropathy.

In NIDDM patients, defining the onset of diabetes is less precise and approximately 5-10% of NIDDM patients have overt nephropathy (proteinuria) at diagnosis. The cumulative incidence of nephropathy in NIDDM is 25% after 20 years duration of the disease. Diabetic

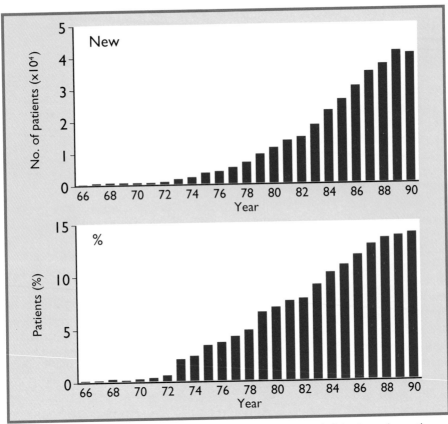

Figure 23 - Patients starting dialysis in Europe with a diagnosis of diabetic nephropathy.

nephropathy is now the single most common cause of end-stage renal failure in the Western world. The majority of patients with diabetes on renal replacement programmes are NIDDM patients, because NIDDM is very much more common than IDDM. The latest reports from the data-base of the European Dialysis and Transplantation Registry (see Figure 23)[1] shows that very many more diabetic patients now receive renal replacement therapy in Europe. The number of patients with a diagnosis of diabetic nephropathy commencing dialysis in Europe increased more than 10-fold in the 15 years up to 1990, and patients with diabetes now form a major proportion of all patients receiving dialysis therapy. This trend does not imply that there has been a sudden rise in the number of cases of diabetic nephropathy; it reflects a general increase in the availability of dialysis, increased referral of patients with diabetes for dialysis and their increased acceptance onto dialysis programmes.

Diabetic nephropathy

Why don't all diabetic patients get nephropathy?

The question as to why only one-quarter to one-third of patients ultimately develop diabetic nephropathy has been at the forefront of debate for a number of years. A logical assumption might be that the diabetic patients who ultimately get nephropathy are those who have had the worst glycaemic control. This is not necessarily the case. Although glycaemic control has an important impact on the likelihood of developing nephropathy, there are many patients with a history of appalling metabolic control who ultimately escape nephropathy, just as there are many with good metabolic control who succumb to nephropathy. Factors other than the quality of glycaemic control are clearly important.

Some studies demonstrate that nephropathy clusters in families, suggesting a possible genetic predisposition. In support of this, Viberti[2] in the UK and Krolewski[3] in the US have suggested that susceptibility to nephropathy is associated with an inherited predisposition to arterial hypertension. These two groups have reported higher blood pressure levels in the parents of diabetic patients with nephropathy compared to parents of normoalbuminuric diabetics. It was subsequently suggested that the cellular basis of this genetic predisposition to hypertension could be defined by demonstrating an increase in red blood cell sodium/lithium countertransport. However, these initial observations have not been confirmed by others, and if there is a genetic predisposition to diabetic nephropathy it does not appear to be acting in a major way via a familial predisposition to hypertension.

More recently, polymorphism of the angiotensin converting enzyme (ACE) gene has been implicated as the genetic factor predisposing to diabetic nephropathy. A deletion polymorphism (DD) of the ACE gene has been associated with an increase in ACE activity in population studies. Alternatively, an insertion polymorphism of the ACE gene (II) has been associated with reduced ACE activity. It has been reported in two studies that DD ACE gene polymorphism is clearly more common in patients with evidence of diabetic nephropathy. This whole field of genetic research, particularly with regard to the ACE genes, is, however, strewn with conflicting data and the observation regarding ACE gene polymorphism and diabetic nephropathy needs evaluating in much larger studies.

There is a complex interplay between established risk factors for diabetic nephropathy, such as blood pressure levels and glycaemic control, and genetic factors that ultimately conspire to determine which patients will succumb to nephropathy. The genetic determinants of this predisposition are presently unknown.

What is microalbuminuria?

Microalbuminuria was first described in the 1960s when Harry Keen in London demonstrated that elevated albumin excretion rates below the level defined as proteinuria (dipstick positive) may have important implications with regard to the natural history of early diabetic renal disease. Microalbuminuria has been used in clinical practice as a marker of progression of renal disease. More recent data suggest that it may also be an important marker of widespread end-organ injury and vascular disease in both IDDM and NIDDM.

In healthy non-diabetic individuals, the normal urinary albumin excretion rate (UAER) is 0-30 mg/24 hours. Clinical proteinuria (positive dipstick test) is usually diagnosed when the UAER exceeds 300 mg/24 hours. A consensus definition for microalbuminuria was obtained in 1986. Microalbuminuria was defined as a urinary albumin excretion rate of >30 mg/24 hours (>20 µg/min) but less than 300 mg/24 hours (<200 µg/min). In other words, it is a sub-clinical increase in urine albumin excretion that would not ordinarily be detected by a conventional urine dipstick test for proteinuria.

Table 14 - Definition of microalbuminuria.

Normal urinary albumin excretion rate (UAER) is <30 mg/24 hours (<20 µg/minute)

Microalbuminuria = UAER of >30 mg/24 hours but <300 mg/24 hours

Proteinuria = UAER sufficient to produce a positive dipstick test for protein

There is tremendous day-to-day variation in urinary albumin excretion because the UAER is influenced, and usually transiently increased, by many factors, such as exercise, posture, fluid loading, dietary protein loading, elevated blood pressure, pregnancy, fever, urinary tract infection and poor glycaemic control, among others. Such factors will produce transient fluctuations in UAER and thus contribute to a normal day-to-day variation in albumin excretion of 40-50%. Moreover, there is a normal diurnal variation whereby the UAER tends to be about 25% higher during the day than during the night. It is not surprising, therefore, that there can be tremendous variation in measurements taken some time apart. For these reasons, any definition of microalbuminuria must take into account the aforementioned factors that can influence the result, and standardised conditions for collection of urine must be applied. Usually the best collection is a timed overnight collection as this has the theoretical advantage of minimising the influence of most of these factors, and is simpler and more convenient for

Diabetic nephropathy

the patient than the traditional 24-hour collection. It is generally agreed that to make a diagnosis of persistent microalbuminuria, the UAER should be in the microalbuminuric range in at least two out of three timed consecutive urine samples, preferably within a six-month period.

How is microalbuminuria measured?

A number of assays are available for the measurement of microalbuminuria; these include radio-immunoassays, immunoturbidimetric or enzyme-linked immunosorbent assays.

Timed urine sample: A timed overnight or 24-hour urine sample is the gold standard for measurement of UAER using any of the aforementioned assay methods. However, in clinical practice, compliance with these collections tends to be poor.

Albumin:creatinine ratio (ACR): A simpler alternative is to analyse an early morning urine sample for the albumin:creatinine ratio. This ratio reduces the influence of urine flow rate and correlates closely with UAER. Our experience with ACR measurements is consistent with that of others and shows that an ACR of greater than 3.0 reliably predicts a UAER of >30 mg/24 hours.

'Bedside' diagnostic tests: Recently, 'bedside' diagnostic testing kits have been developed. The Micral-test (Boehringer Mannheim, Germany) and the Nycocard U-Albumin test (Nycomed Pharma AS, Oslo, Norway) are both simple and rapid; they record concentrations of albumin ranging from 0-100 g/ml for the Micral-test and 10-160 g/ml for the Nycocard test. These tests are robust, sensitive and specific, and provide an instant 'bedside' result.

Recommendations for screening and monitoring of microalbuminuria

The recent St. Vincent Declaration Action Programme[4] recommended that all patients with IDDM who are over 12 years old (microalbuminuria is very rare before puberty), and have had the disease for at least five years, should be screened. Moreover, all NIDDM patients should be screened from the time of diagnosis. This screening for microalbuminuria should take place at least once a year until the age of 70 years. Although timed urine collections are recommended, determination of ACR from an early morning urine sample is satisfactory for screening. Figure 24 shows an example of a screening programme for microalbuminuria that could be applied simply in clinical practice. In this schema, patients are initially screened using an ACR measurement or a bedside diagnostic test for microalbumin levels using their first-morning-urine sample. An ACR of <3.0 or a urine albumin concentration of <20 mg/l (this approximates to <30 mg/24 hrs, assuming a daily urine output of 1.5 litres) is considered normal and the patients are then retested annually.

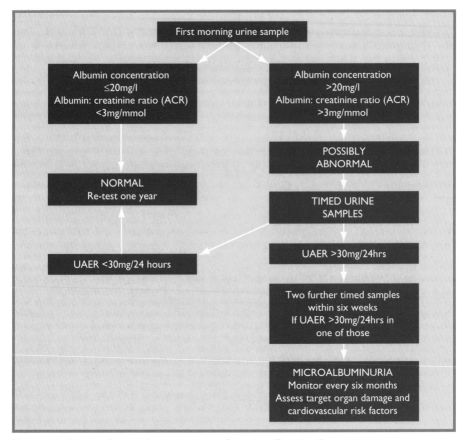

First morning urine sample

Albumin concentration
≤20mg/l
Albumin: creatinine ratio (ACR)
<3mg/mmol

Albumin concentration
>20mg/l
Albumin: creatinine ratio (ACR)
>3mg/mmol

POSSIBLY
ABNORMAL

NORMAL
Re-test one year

TIMED URINE
SAMPLES

UAER <30mg/24 hours

UAER >30mg/24hrs

Two further timed samples
within six weeks
If UAER >30mg/24hrs in
one of those

MICROALBUMINURIA
Monitor every six months
Assess target organ damage and
cardiovascular risk factors

Figure 24 - Proposed screening programme for microalbuminuria.

If the test is abnormal, then the UAER should be measured formally in a timed sample. If the UAER is then found to be <30 mg/24 hours in the timed sample, the patient is returned to the annual screening programme. If the UAER is >30 mg/24 hours, two further timed urine samples are tested within six weeks. If one of these further tests confirms an elevated UAER (>30 mg/24 hours) the patient has microalbuminuria. Microalbuminuric patients should then undergo a formal evaluation to assess their degree of target organ damage and CV risk factors. They should probably have their UAER measured every six months thereafter. The objective of this screening strategy is to identify the sub-group of diabetic patients who are at much higher risk for the development of hypertension, renal disease, retinopathy, neuropathy and CV disease in general.

Diabetic nephropathy

The cost of such a screening strategy must of course be set against the potential benefit of treatment. A recent preliminary analysis indicates that any therapeutic intervention that has an effect in more than 8% of patients would produce a positive cost:benefit ratio, thus justifying screening.

Risk factors for the development of microalbuminuria

To define the risk factors associated with the development of persistent microalbuminuria in non-microalbuminuric, normotensive IDDM patients, a four-year prospective study was recently undertaken by the Microalbuminuria Collaborative Study Group in the UK[5]. Of the 137 patients studied, 11 developed microalbuminuria. The patients who progressed to microalbuminuria tended to have higher systolic and diastolic blood pressures, higher baseline UAER and poorer glycaemic control at baseline, and were more likely to be smokers. Blood pressure and smoking were identified as independent determinants for the development of microalbuminuira (see Table 15)[5]. These results confirm the conclusions reached in other studies, notably that elevated blood pressure, poor glycaemic control and a history of smoking are all associated with the development of nephropathy and other vascular complications of diabetes. The importance of rigorous glycaemic control was confirmed by the recent Diabetes Control and Complications Trial research group (DCCT)[6], which showed that very strict glycaemic control (to levels probably not achievable in normal clinical practice) reduced the risk of progressing from a normal albumin excretion rate to microalbuminuria by 39% and decreased the risk of progression from microalbuminuria to proteinuria by 54%. However, other studies have shown that once overt proteinuria is established, strict glycaemic control has no beneficial effect on the progressive increase in urine protein excretion.

Similar associations with microalbuminuria have been reported for NIDDM. In a five-year prospective study of NIDDM patients in Japan, approximately 30% of patients developed microalbuminuria, and the most predictive factors were higher mean blood pressure at baseline and blood

Table 15 - The factors associated with the development of microalbuminuria in a prospective study of IDDM and NIDDM patients (* = most strongly predictive).

- Elevated systolic and/or diastolic blood pressure*
- Poor glycaemic control
- High baseline urinary albumin excretion rate*
- Smoking

pressure that progressively increased as microalbuminuria developed. Poor diabetic control was also predictive, but had a lesser impact than blood pressure.

The significance of microalbuminuria in IDDM

Once microalbuminuira becomes established, there is a tendency for the patient to develop a progressive year-on-year rise in UAER (approximately a 20% increase in UAER per year) until eventually the patient develops proteinuria (see Figure 25). The progressive rise in UAER is paralleled by a progressive rise in blood pressure, so that by the time proteinuria has developed a majority of the patients are hypertensive[7]. There are wide variations in the estimates of the prevalence of microalbuminuria in IDDM patients. Early studies suggested a prevalence of 18-30%; more recent studies have suggested a lower prevalence of 9-14%. The annual rate of progression from normoalbuminuria to microalbuminuria in IDDM patients is approximately 3% and occurs in those individuals with the high risk profile shown in Table 15. It used to be said that persistent microalbuminuria predicts the development of proteinuria and nephropathy in approximately 80% of IDDM patients. However, more recent studies suggest that progression from microalbuminuria to proteinuria (nephropathy) occurs in 20-40% of IDDM patients. Moreover, the prognostic significance of microalbuminuria may be less ominous when detected in patients who have had IDDM for more than 20 years.

Thus, the development of microalbuminuria is powerfully predictive for the development of nephropathy, but it must also be emphasised that microalbuminuria is also associated with the development of other diabetic complications, most notably microangiopathy and CV disease.

The significance of microalbuminuria in NIDDM

In NIDDM patients, microalbuminuria also predicts the development of proteinuria and clinical nephropathy, but it is much more predictive of a premature death from CV disease. The prevalence of microalbuminuria in NIDDM has been less well defined than in IDDM. Various studies suggest that microalbuminuria is detectable in 20-35% of patients at the time of diagnosis of NIDDM. Cross-sectional studies of patients with established NIDDM yield microalbuminuria prevalence rates of 10-50%. Microalbuminuria predicts the development of proteinuria in approximately 20% of NIDDM patients. The development of clinical nephropathy and subsequent renal failure appears to be a less prominent consequence than in IDDM patients. This is because microalbuminuria in NIDDM patients is so strongly predictive of morbidity and early mortality from CV disease. Various studies have demonstrated that even a small degree of microalbuminuria predicts a considerable increase in the mortality of NIDDM patients even during short observation periods. Thus,

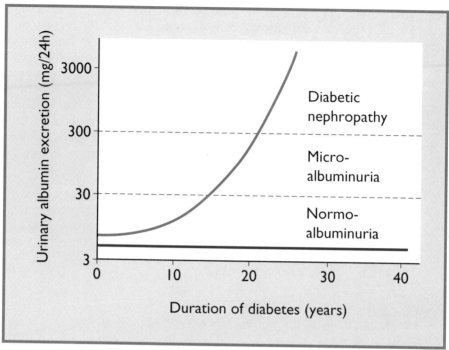

Figure 25 - Urinary albumin excretion in relation to duration of diabetes in IDDM patients with and without development of diabetic nephropathy. Microalbuminuria is defined as urinary albumin excretion exceeding the normal limit but below the level for clinical nephropathy (30-300 mg/24-hour).

the development of microalbuminuria in NIDDM patients is particularly ominous and such patients will often die from CV disease before sufficient time has elapsed to allow clinical nephropathy to develop.

Microalbuminuria is not just a marker of renal disease

The significance of microalbuminuria and proteinuria in diabetic patients extends beyond the kidney. The development of microalbuminuria in IDDM and NIDDM and its subsequent progression to proteinuria identifies a subgroup of diabetic patients who are at grave risk for the accelerated development of microvascular and macrovascular disease that will ultimately predispose to considerable morbidity and premature death.

Microalbuminuria, proteinuria and diabetic microvascular disease

Retinopathy

An association between clinical diabetic nephropathy and the development of proliferative retinopathy has long been recognised. IDDM patients with proteinuria have an 8 to 10 times higher annual incidence of proliferative

---

Diabetic nephropathy

retinopathy than IDDM patients without proteinuria (Figure 26)[8]. The annual incidence of proliferative retinopathy in those with established proteinuria was 12%, whereas in those without proteinuria there was a low, constant annual incidence rate of one to two per cent. However, further analysis of Figure 26 shows that there was a steep increase in the annual incidence of proliferative retinopathy 5 to 10 years before clinical nephropathy (proteinuria) was identified. Thus, it can be confidently assumed that this accelerated phase of microvascular injury occurred during the period of time when microalbuminuria was developing in these patients. This conclusion is supported by the observation that an increased UAER in diabetic patients is associated with an increased prevalence of blindness (see Figure 27).

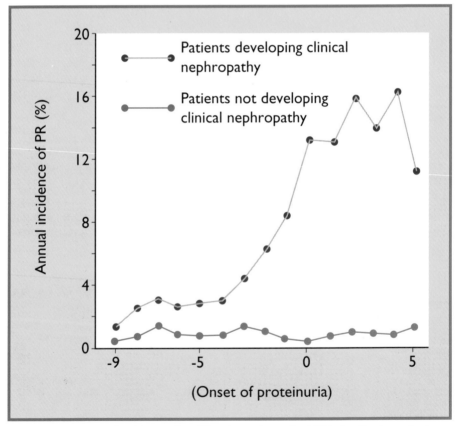

Figure 26 - The annual incidence of proliferative retinopathy (PR) in insulin-dependent diabetic patients developing clinical nephropathy, and patients not developing clinical nephropathy.

Neuropathy

Diabetic neuropathy is also commonly associated with clinical nephropathy (proteinuria). Moreover, just as for retinopathy, the prevalence of neuropathy is correlated with the magnitude of the increase in UAER (see Figure 27)[9]. These observations suggest that there is also accelerated development of diabetic neuropathy during the microalbuminuric phase of diabetes.

Cardiomyopathy

Cardiomyopathy is another important microvascular complication of diabetes. A recent cross-sectional study used maximal aerobic work capacity as an index of cardiac function in IDDM patients. IDDM patients without an

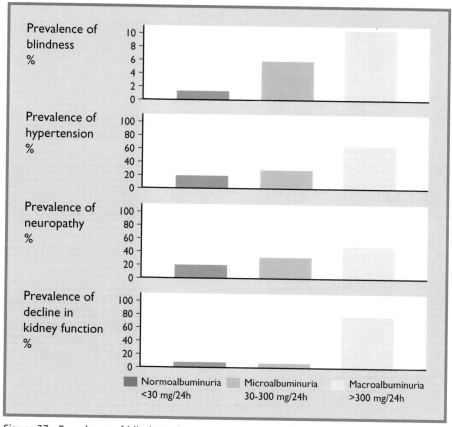

Figure 27 - Prevalence of blindness, hypertension, neuropathy and reduced kidney function in IDDM patients with normoalbuminuria (30 mg/24 hours), microalbuminuria (30-300 mg/24 hours) and macroalbuminuria (300 mg/24 hours).

Diabetic nephropathy

increase in UAER had similar maximal aerobic work capacities to non-diabetic subjects. In contrast, IDDM patients with clinical nephropathy (proteinuria) had a 40% reduction in their cardiac performance (see Figure 28)[10]. What is more alarming is that this defect in cardiac function had already developed during the microalbuminuric phase of their disease (Figure 28)[10]. Further studies using radionucleotide cardiac imaging revealed that this deficit in performance was explained by a reduction in stroke volume and cardiac output at rest and during exercise in the patients with an increased UAER.

These observations and clinical experience suggest that even slight increases in UAER in diabetic patients are associated with a progressive rise in blood pressure and the widespread development of microvascular disease. Moreover, microalbuminuria appears to identify a phase of accelerated microvascular injury.

Microalbuminuria, proteinuria and diabetic macrovascular disease

IDDM patients
There is a close association between the development of proteinuria and CV disease in diabetic patients. In a case-controlled study of 118 young IDDM patients, the cumulative incidence of CHD was 40% in patients with proteinuria

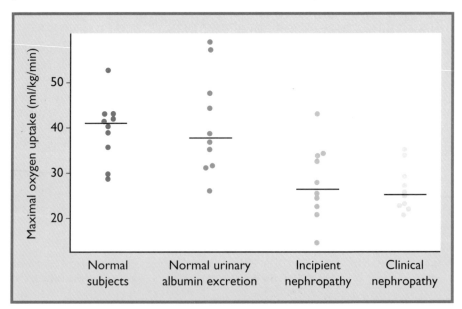

Figure 28 - Maximal oxygen uptake in normal subjects and insulin-dependent diabetic patients with normal urinary albumin excretion (<30 mg/24 hours); incipient nephropathy (urinary albumin excretion in the range of 30-300 mg/24 hours). Horizontal bars indicate median values.

Diabetic nephropathy

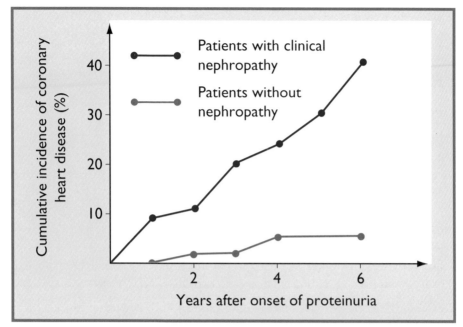

Figure 29 - *The cumulative incidence of major electrocardiographic abnormalities and clinical coronary heart disease in insulin-dependent diabetic patients with clinical nephropathy, and patients without clinical nephropathy. The two groups were followed to the same age and diabetes duration.*

during a six-year follow-up, compared to a rate of only 5% in those without proteinuria (see Figure 29)[11]. The impact of increased UAER on CV disease in IDDM was further emphasised in a much larger study comprising 2,890 patients[12]. The overall mortality from CV disease in IDDM patients without proteinuria was 4.2 times that of the general non-diabetic population. However, the CV mortality of IDDM patients with proteinuria was astonishingly high, 37 times that of the general population. The impact of an increased UAER on CV morbidity and mortality is striking in IDDM, but less apparent than that observed in NIDDM patients.

NIDDM patients
It is now generally accepted that microalbuminuria is the most potent risk factor for mortality in NIDDM patients, and that this increase in mortality is due to CV disease. In a prospective study of 211 NIDDM patients followed for eight to nine years, UAER was the best predictor of long-term mortality (see Table 16)[13].

In another prospective study of 141 NIDDM patients[14], the excess mortality was significantly increased in those with microalbuminuria (28%)

Table 16 - Impact of UAER on mortality in NIDDM. Number of deaths in 211 NIDDM patients according to their quartiles of urinary albumin excretion (*χ^2 = 21.4, p<0.0001).

Quartiles	1	2	3	4
UAER (mg/24 hrs)	<11.4	11.4 - 25.0	25.1 - 112.2	≥112.2
Number of deaths				
Observed*	21	18	26	37
Expected*	29	28	27	19

compared to those without microalbuminuria (4%), even though the study was only of short duration (3.4 years). Moreover, the predictive power of microalbuminuria persisted after adjustment for other major risk factors. Finally, in a follow-up study of 175 NIDDM patients with microalbuminuria[15], 120 (68%) had died within 10 years. Of those deaths, 58% were due to CV disease whereas only 7% were due to renal disease. Thus, microalbuminuria is very powerfully predictive of premature death in NIDDM patients and the cause of death in the vast majority of these cases will be CV disease rather than renal disease.

The significance of microalbuminuria in the non-diabetic population

The association between an increase in UAER and the likelihood of suffering premature morbidity and mortality related to CV disease is also strong in the non-diabetic general population. In a study of 187 non-diabetic subjects over the age of 40 years attending a community screening programme in Islington, London, the prevalence of CHD was 33% in those with a normal UAER and 74% in those with microalbuminuria. The prevalence of peripheral vascular disease and the subsequent risk of death was also markedly increased in those individuals with a UAER in the microalbuminuric range (see Table 17)[16]. Similarly, non-diabetic hypertensive patients experience a much higher CV morbidity if they have proteinuria when compared to hypertensive patients without an increased UAER (see Figure 30)[17].

Diabetic nephropathy

Table 17 - The impact of the presence of microalbuminuria on the subsequent development of cardiovascular disease in non-diabetic subjects over the age of 40 years studied for almost four years.		
	Normal UAER	**Microalbuminuria**
Ischaemic heart disease	33%	74%
Peripheral vascular disease	9.7%	44%
Death	2%	33%

Why does microalbuminuria predict generalised vascular disease?
It is clear from the evidence cited above that microalbuminuria in diabetic patients is not just a marker of renal disease but is a strong predictor of a more generalised vascular injury. It is now evident that patients developing microalbuminuria also develop in tandem a constellation of risk factors for CV disease (see Chapter 4). This suggests a common pathogenetic mechanism in the development of microalbuminuria and atherosclerosis.

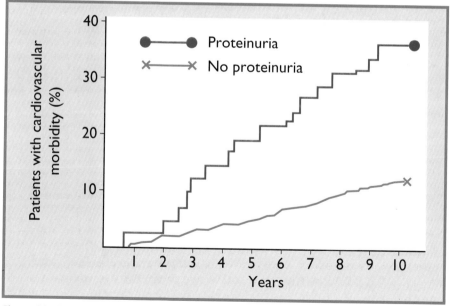

Figure 30 - Ten-year cumulative incidence of cardiovascular morbidity in patients with proteinuria at initial examination (n=41) compared with patients free from proteinuria (n=643). According to the life table method of analysis p<0.001.

Endothelial dysfunction

Increased permeability to circulating macromolecules such as albumin is one of the earliest events in the pathogenesis of vascular injury. Diabetic patients with microalbuminuria exhibit a generalised increase in vascular permeability to albumin. In this regard, microalbuminuria in diabetic patients represents a subtle early marker of a generalised vascular injury. In support of this, an increased UAER in diabetic patients is invariably associated with increased circulating levels of Von Willebrand factor, a factor released by the endothelium in response to injury (see Chapter 4).

Clotting abnormalities

Abnormalities in blood clotting generating a pro-thrombotic tendency are also more common in diabetic patients with an increased UAER. These abnormalities include:

- increased fibrinogen turnover and increased plasma fibrinogen levels,
- impaired tissue plasminogen response to exercise, and
- changes in platelet function leading to increased platelet adhesion.

Lipid abnormalities

In NIDDM, various studies have highlighted a link between microalbuminuria and the magnitude of insulin resistance. A cross-sectional study of IDDM patients also concluded that those patients with evidence of insulin resistance were more likely to be microalbuminuric. As microalbuminuria is associated with a broad constellation of CV risk factors (see Chapter 4), this link may also be relevant to the link between an increased UAER and CV disease. In addition, lipoprotein (a) levels are also raised in diabetic patients with increased UAER.

Abnormal blood pressure regulation

In IDDM there is compelling evidence that blood pressure regulation is abnormal at the time of onset of microalbuminuria. Evidence is also emerging to suggest that blood pressure regulation is abnormal in NIDDM patients with microalbuminuria (see Chapter 2). Thus, diabetic patients with microalbuminuria are likely to have higher blood pressures than those with a normal albumin excretion.

Left ventricular hypertrophy (LVH)

Echocardiographic studies of diabetic patients with microalbuminuria and apparently normal 'office' blood pressures have revealed early evidence of LVH. Increased left ventricular mass is usually an adaptive response to an elevated blood pressure. The development of LVH in microalbuminuric patients is further evidence of the abnormally high 24-hour blood pressure load in these patients. LVH is an ominous development in hypertensive patients as it is strongly predictive of premature CV morbidity and mortality.

Left ventricular dysfunction
Microalbuminuria is associated with evidence of left ventricular dysfunction (Figure 23). This will ultimately predispose to heart failure and contribute to an excess CV morbidity and mortality.

Microalbuminuria: an important surrogate for accelerated vascular injury
The aforementioned data suggest that the onset of microalbuminuria is an ominous development in diabetic patients. Microalbuminuria is much more than a marker of diabetic nephropathy. Microalbuminuria is an important surrogate for abnormal blood pressure regulation and CV disease risk-factor clustering. Screening for microalbuminuria in clinical practice will help to identify a subgroup of IDDM and NIDDM patients who are at grave risk of developing microvascular and macrovascular disease. In so doing, it will alert the physician to the need to be particularly vigilant in screening for established target organ damage and in managing the patient's blood pressure, glycaemic control and other modifiable CV risk factors.

REFERENCES

1. Raine AEG, Margreiter R *et al*. Report on management of renal failure in Europe XXII 1991. *Nephrol Dial Transp* 1992; **2**: 7-35.

2. Mangili R, Bending JJ, Scott G, Li LK, Gupta A, Viberti GC. Increased sodium-lithium countertransport activity in red cells of patients with insulin-dependent diabetes and nephropathy. *N Engl J Med* 1988; **318**: 146-50.

3. Krolewski AS, Canessa M, Warram JH, Laffel LMB, Christlieb AR, Knowler WC, Rand LI. Predisposition to hypertension and susceptibility to renal disease in insulin-dependent diabetes mellitus. *N Engl J Med* 1988; **318**: 140-5.

4. Krans HMJ, Porta M, Keen H (eds). Guidelines for the prevention of renal failure. In: *Diabetes care and research in Europe: The St Vincent Declaration action programme*. WHO Regional Office for Europe, 1992: 29-32.

5. Microalbuminuria Collaborative Study Group, United Kingdom. Risk factors for development of microalbuminuria in insulin dependent diabetic patients: a cohort study. *Br Med J* 1993; **306**: 1235-9.

6. The Diabetes Control and Complications Trial Research Group. The effect of intensive treatment of diabetes on the development and progression of long-term complications in insulin-dependent diabetes mellitus. *N Engl J Med* 1993; **329**: 977-8.

7. Mathiesen ER *et al*. Relationship between blood pressure and urinary albumin excretion in development of microalbuminuria. *Diabetes* 1990; **39**: 245-9.

8. Kofoed-Enevoldsen A, Jensen T, Borch-Johnsen K, Deckert T. Incidence of retinopathy in type 1 (insulin-dependent) diabetes: association with clinical nephropathy. *J Diabetes Compl* 1987; **1**: 96-9.

9. Parving H-H *et al*. Prevalence of microalbuminuria, arterial hypertension, retinopathy and neuropathy in insulin dependent diabetes. *Br Med J* 1988; **296**: 156-60.

10. Jensen T, Richter EA, Feldt-Rasmussen B, Kelbæk H, Deckert T. Impaired aerobic work capacity in insulin-dependent diabetics with increased urinary albumin excretion. *Br Med J* 1988; **296**: 1352-4.

11. Jensen T, Borch-Johnsen K, Kofoed-Enevoldsen A, Deckert T. Coronary heart disease in young type 1 (insulin-dependent) diabetic patients with and without diabetic nephropathy: incidence and risk factors. *Diabetologia* 1987; **30**: 144-8.

12. Borch-Johnsen K, Kreiner S. Proteinuria: value as predictor of cardiovascular mortality in insulin dependent diabetes mellitus. *Br Med J* 1987; **294**: 1651-4.

13. Damsgaard EM et al. Eight to nine year mortality in known non-insulin dependent diabetics and controls. *Kidney Int* 1992; **41**: 731-5.

14. Mattock MB *et al*. Prospective study of microalbuminuria as predictor of mortality in NIDDM. *Diabetes* 1992; **41**: 736-41.

15. Schmitz A, Vaeth M. Microalbuminuria: a major risk factor in non-insulin-dependent diabetes. A 10-year follow-up study of 503 patients. *Diabet Med* 1988; **5**: 126-34.

16. Yudkin JS, Forrest RD, Jackson CA. Microalbuminuria as predictor of vascular disease in non-diabetic subjects: Islington Diabetes Survey. *Lancet* 1988; **ii**: 530-3.

17. Samuelsson O *et al*. Predictors of cardiovascular morbidity in treated hypertension: results from the primary prevention trial in Göteborg, Sweden. *J Hypertens* 1985; **3**: 167-76.

CHAPTER 5 - SUMMARY POINTS

- Diabetic nephropathy is defined clinically as the 'triad' of hypertension, proteinuria and declining renal function.
- Persistent microalbuminuria predicts the development of nephropathy in IDDM patients.
- Persistent microalbuminuria also predicts the development of nephropathy in NIDDM patients, but is more strongly predictive of a premature death from CV disease.
- Annual screening of diabetic subjects for microalbuminuria is cost effective and its presence identifies a high-risk group.
- Patients with persistent microalbuminuria should be screened for target organ damage and have their CV risk factors, including hypertension, managed aggressively.
- Microalbuminuria is not just a marker of renal disease.
- Microalbuminuria predicts the development of widespread microvascular disease in diabetic subjects.
- Microalbuminuria is also predictive of premature CV morbidity and mortality in non-diabetic subjects.

Chapter Six

EVALUATION OF THE DIABETIC PATIENT WITH HYPERTENSION

The problem of defining hypertension in diabetic patients

The optimal blood pressure for IDDM and NIDDM patients is not known. Moreover, the level of blood pressure at which therapeutic intervention should be considered in diabetic patients has not been defined. One of the enduring problems has been the lack of data regarding the efficacy of antihypertensive therapy in diabetic patients. It is remarkable that no large, population-based, randomised trials of antihypertensive therapy have been conducted in diabetic patients. This is even more remarkable when one considers the enormous impact of hypertension on cardiovascular (CV) morbidity and mortality in diabetic patients. This paucity of data is further compounded by the fact that diabetic patients have frequently been excluded from the large, prospective trials of antihypertensive therapy. Moreover, in the few large-scale clinical trials that have enrolled people with diabetes in appreciable numbers, much of the information regarding the outcome of the diabetic cohort has not been reported. In two such recent large clinical trials, 10% of the hypertensive participants were also diabetic and limited data from the diabetic sub-groups have been reported:

Hypertension Detection and Follow-up Program (HDFP)[1]

Ten per cent of the participants in this trial had a fasting blood glucose level ≥7.8 mmol/l or were taking medication for diabetes. The beneficial effect of diuretic-based stepped care antihypertensive therapy on total mortality was similar in the diabetic cohort when compared to the whole group. Data regarding cardiovascular endpoints in the diabetic sub-group have not been reported.

Systolic Hypertension in the Elderly Program (SHEP)[2]

Ten per cent of the participants in this clinical trial were diabetic. This trial examined the effects of thiazide diuretic-based antihypertensive therapy on the primary end-point of stroke. In the diabetic sub-group the relative risk reductions on antihypertensive therapy for all major end-points (fatal or non-fatal stroke, coronary heart disease death or non-fatal myocardial infarction, all major cardiovascular events and total mortality) were similar to those of the whole group.

It should be noted that neither of the aforementioned trials was designed specifically to address the impact of diabetes on the efficacy of antihypertensive therapy in reducing cardiovascular morbidity and mortality. Nevertheless, these limited data do suggest that the treatment of hypertension in diabetic patients is likely to be at least as effective at reducing the risk of cardiovascular events as it is in the non-diabetic population. Based on this important assumption, and despite the aforementioned limitations, various consensus reports have emanated from around the world with the aim of providing guidelines on the management of hypertension in diabetic patients.

Guidelines on the guidelines

Few countries have produced specific guidelines for hypertension management in diabetic patients, and the guidelines adopted for the management of hypertension tend to be those designed for the population in general. In many early studies of diabetic patients, the World Health Organisation (WHO) definition of hypertension was usually used to categorise patients.

The WHO, in 1978, defined a normal adult blood pressure as ≤140/90 mmHg (DBP measured at phase V of ≤90 mmHg). Hypertension in adults was arbitrarily defined as a SBP ≥160 mmHg and/or DBP ≥95 mmHg. The term 'borderline' was used to denote blood pressure values between the normal and hypertensive ranges.

The first nationally-endorsed guidelines for the management of hypertension that specifically targeted diabetic patients were produced in the US and were updated very recently. The *USA National high blood pressure education programme working group report on hypertension in diabetes* defined hypertension in diabetic patients as a SBP ≥140 mmHg and/or a DBP ≥90 mmHg[3]. This report did not suggest different thresholds for IDDM and NIDDM subjects. The recommended treatment goal was to maintain blood pressure levels at less than 130/85 mmHg.

In the UK, the British Hypertension Society (BHS) issued guidelines in 1993 for the management of hypertension[4]. These guidelines were directed at the general population and did not differentiate between diabetic and non-diabetic patients. In these guidelines, the threshold for the treatment of hypertension was SBP ≥160 mmHg and/or DBP ≥100 mmHg. The guidelines did, however, suggest that the diastolic threshold should be reduced to 90 mmHg in the presence of other CV risk factors or evidence of target organ damage. This latter statement would thus qualify diabetic patients for treatment at this lower diastolic threshold of ≥90 mmHg as diabetes *per se* is an additional CV risk factor. The treatment goal stated in the BHS guidelines was to reduce DBP to below 90 mmHg and although no firm recommendations were made, it was considered prudent to maintain SBP below 160 mmHg.

In 1994, Professor Harry Keen (Guy's Hospital, London) convened a working party in the UK to produce specific guidelines for the management of hypertension in diabetic patients. These guidelines suggested different blood pressure thresholds for intervention in IDDM and NIDDM patients.

Table 18 - Comparison of the intervention thresholds for blood pressure treatment in the guidelines issued by the World Health Organisation (WHO), the British Hypertension Society (BHS), the USA Working Party on Hypertension in Diabetes (USA) and a UK Working Party on Diabetes and Hypertension (UKWP) which issued different recommendations for IDDM and NIDDM. The BHS guidelines suggest a diastolic blood pressure of 100 mmHg for intervention in general but 90 mmHg in those with additional cardiovascular risk factors, e.g. diabetes.

	Diastolic BP	Systolic BP	Treatment goal
WHO	95	160	<140/90
BHS	90-100+	160	<160/90
USA	90	140	<130/85
UKWP (IDDM)	90	140	<140/90
UKWP (NIDDM)	90	160	<160/90

For IDDM patients it defined hypertension as a blood pressure $\geq 140/90$ mmHg, a view consistent with the current US guidelines. For NIDDM patients these guidelines defined hypertension as $\geq 160/90$ mmHg. Moreover, it was recommended that if the blood pressure was $\geq 140/90$ mmHg, but $\leq 160/90$ mmHg, in NIDDM patients (i.e. 'borderline hypertension' in NIDDM), non-pharmacological advice would be appropriate in an attempt to lower blood pressure and modify associated CV risk factors. The treatment goal suggested by these guidelines was to reduce and maintain diastolic blood pressure below 90 mmHg. Although no specific recommendations were made regarding the treatment goal for SBP, the assumption is that they be maintained below the intervention threshold. The aforementioned guidelines are compared in Table 18.

Towards a consensus from available guidelines

Blood pressure thresholds for treatment intervention
Dogmatic recommendations for the management of hypertension in diabetic patients are not possible due to the lack of trial data. Nevertheless, one can reasonably assume that blood pressure control should be at least as aggressive in diabetic patients as it is in the non-diabetic population. Moreover, one can define the points of agreement from various guidelines

Table 19 - Towards a consensus from available guidelines.			
Patient	Threshold systolic BP mmHg	Threshold diastolic BP mmHg	Target for treated BP mmHg
IDDM ± target organ damage	≥140	≥90	≤140/90
NIDDM + target organ damage	≥140	≥90	≤140/90
NIDDM - no target organ damage	≥160	≥90	≤160/90 (≤140/90 if poss.)

(see Table 19). From the guidelines given above, there is an emerging consensus regarding the intervention threshold for diastolic blood pressure, i.e. ≥90 mmHg. There is also agreement that a SBP ≥160 mmHg is undesirable. The US guidelines have taken a more aggressive stance with regard to the SBP threshold, i.e. ≥ 140 mmHg. Although there are no trial data to support this recommendation, it is not unreasonable when one considers the epidemiological associations between elevated blood pressures and microvascular and macrovascular disease (see Chapter 3). Thus, in patients with IDDM, this lower SBP threshold, i.e. ≥140 mmHg, does seem appropriate, and where other CV risk factors co-exist or there is target organ damage (including microalbuminuria) it is my view that this threshold would certainly indicate the need for therapy. The US guidelines suggest a similar systolic threshold (140 mmHg) for IDDM and NIDDM patients, whereas other guidelines have accepted a higher SBP threshold of 160 mmHg for NIDDM patients. The recent UK working party approach was a compromise in this area, recommending treatment at SBP ≥140 mmHg if target organ damage is present or 160 mmHg if not.

Treated blood pressure goals
The effectiveness of antihypertensive therapy in terms of reducing cardiovascular morbidity and mortality is entirely dependent on the quality of blood pressure control. Achieving and maintaining a diastolic blood pressure below 90 mmHg is recommended by all guidelines. A systolic pressure of less than 140 mmHg would seem to be a prudent target in all treated IDDM patients. In NIDDM, a treated SBP of less than 140 mmHg should be the goal in all patients and in particular those with evidence of target organ damage. This may not be easy to achieve in NIDDM patients and a treated SBP of less than 160 mmHg would be an acceptable goal in NIDDM patients

without target organ damage. This view was shared by a recent European NIDDM policy group working under sponsorship of the International Diabetes Foundation. This policy group issued a desktop guide for the management of NIDDM which suggested that ≤140/90 mmHg represented good control of blood pressure in NIDDM patients.

Blood pressure measurement

- Blood pressure should initially be measured in both arms with the patient supine or seated.

- The cuff bladder size should be appropriate for the patient, i.e. larger cuff size in obese patients; using a standard cuff size in obese patients leads to an overestimation of blood pressure.

- The diastolic blood pressure is recorded at the disappearance of sound (phase V).

- Record all blood pressure readings to the nearest 2 mmHg; rounding up to the nearest 10 is not acceptable.

- Record a standing as well as a supine or sitting blood pressure because of the common occurrence of orthostatic hypotension in diabetic patients.

- Record at least two separate blood pressure readings at each visit.

- Hypertension should not be diagnosed on the basis of measurements at a single clinic visit.

- Record blood pressure readings on four or more separate visits to define the blood pressure threshold and confirm or exclude the presence of hypertension.

- The length of time for observation will depend on the severity of the hypertension. Patients with mild hypertension and no evidence of target organ injury can be observed over three to six months.

- In more severe hypertension, or those with target organ damage, the assessment will take place over a much shorter period of time.

- All patients with diabetes should have their blood pressure measured at each clinic visit, and at least annually.

Clinical evaluation of the hypertensive diabetic patient

The clinical evaluation of the hypertensive patient with diabetes should endeavour to determine:

- whether there are any potentially curable causes of the hypertension;

- the severity of the hypertension;

- whether there are associated cardiovascular risk factors;
- the extent of target organ injury;
- the quality of the patient's glycaemic control.

Hypertension must be viewed as an important, but not exclusive, component of the patient's overall cardiovascular risk. A comprehensive assessment of the hypertensive diabetic subject is essential to quantify the risk accurately, identify remediable risk factors and tailor the selection of any drug therapy to meet the needs of that individual.

Key points in medical history

- Family history of hypertension, diabetes, renal disease and cardiovascular disease.
- Patient's history of renal disease, retinopathy and cardiovascular disease.
- Duration of diabetes and duration of hypertension.
- History of medication, including drugs that may induce hypertension (see below).
- Lifestyle; i.e. smoking, alcohol intake, exercise levels, obesity, diet.

Drug therapies that may elevate blood pressure

This list is not exclusive, but serves to highlight common drug therapies that may also influence blood pressure levels and the patient's response to antihypertensive therapy.

Oral contraceptives

All women taking the oral contraceptive pill experience a rise in blood pressure. This is usually insignificant. However, in approximately 5% of women, this small rise may elevate a blood pressure reading already at the upper end of the normal range, into the abnormal range. There is no evidence to suggest that the oral contraceptive pill-induced rise in blood pressure is any greater in diabetic subjects. On the subject of female hormones, women with normal blood pressures on treatment or with blood pressures in the high normal range should not be denied the potential benefits of hormone replacement therapy.

Oral corticosteroids

High-dose steroid therapy elevates blood pressure. The effect of lower-dose corticosteroids, such as those used to treat asthma, is less predictable.

Carbenoxolone/liquorice
Carbenoxolone-based drugs were used until recently to treat peptic ulcer disease and can elevate blood pressure. Liquorice itself when eaten in large quantities can also elevate blood pressure.

Anorectic drugs and cold cures
These remedies often contain sympathomimetic drugs that can elevate blood pressure.

Non-steroidal anti-inflammatory drugs (NSAIDs)
These agents promote salt and water retention and can elevate blood pressure. They can also block the antihypertensive actions of thiazide diuretics and blunt the action of ACE inhibitors, some vasodilators and beta-blockers. The calcium antagonists do not appear to be affected by NSAIDs.

Physical examination of the hypertensive diabetic patient
A physical examination is performed to determine whether there is any evidence to suggest an underlying, potentially curable cause for hypertension, the nature and extent of any target organ damage, and to identify factors that may influence the selection of drug therapy for hypertension. The physical examination should include the following:

- Measurement of height and weight and also the waist-to-hip ratio to give an index of obesity and body fat distribution.

- The general examination should look for evidence of endocrine disorders that may co-exist and contribute to the development of diabetes and hypertension, e.g. Cushing's disease. Also look for signs of hyperlipidaemia.

- At least two blood pressure measurements during the clinic visit, measurements from both arms and measurements in standing and supine positions are required to define whether there are significant changes in postural blood pressure. A wide arm blood pressure cuff must be used for patients with obese arms.

- Peripheral pulses should be examined to determine whether they are present, absent or diminished.

- The carotid arteries and femoral arteries are examined for arterial bruits.

- Look for evidence of radio-femoral delay. Normally the radial and femoral pulses are synchronous. If there is a delay in the femoral pulse relative to the radial pulse, this may indicate the presence of an aortic coarctation; if the coarctation is severe, the femoral pulses may be absent. It should be noted, however, that in older patients with hypertension, absent femoral pulses are most commonly due to atherosclerosis.

- The heart should be carefully examined to define whether there is clinical evidence of left ventricular hypertrophy or enlargement, murmurs, arrhythmias and S3 and S4 heart sounds.

- The patient's fluid status should be carefully assessed, determining whether there is evidence of fluid overload, i.e. peripheral oedema, raised jugular venous pressure or evidence of pulmonary oedema.

- The abdomen should be examined for renal masses, i.e. polycystic kidneys or a downward displaced kidney due to an adrenal mass. Is there evidence of an abdominal aortic aneurysm? Are renal bruits audible? Renal bruits are often best heard a few centimetres either side of the umbilicus. Where renal impairment is known to be present, the abdomen should also be examined for the presence of a bladder which may be enlarged due to neuropathic disease or prostatic enlargement.

- Funduscopy should be performed and retinal photographs are especially useful, where the technology is available, to define the extent of hypertensive and diabetic retinopathy.

- A neurological assessment is important to document evidence of neuropathy, especially peripheral sensory and vibratory deficits.

- The urine should be examined by a dipstick test for blood and protein, and assayed for microalbumin levels.

Physical and simple laboratory findings suggesting secondary hypertension

- Palpable kidneys (i.e. polycystic kidneys or adrenal mass).

- Renal bruits (i.e. renovascular disease).

- Delayed or absent femoral pulses (i.e. aortic coarctation).

- Truncal obesity, pigmented striae (i.e. Cushing's syndrome).

- Paroxysmal tachycardia, hypertension, sweating (i.e. phaeochromocytoma).

- Haematuria and proteinuria (i.e. possibly non-diabetic renal disease).

- Hypokalaemia on no medication (i.e. hyperaldosteronism).

Investigation of diabetic subjects with hypertension

Further investigation of the hypertensive diabetic patient is required to:

- Establish whether there are co-existing risk factors for cardiovascular disease, e.g. dyslipidaemia.
- Define the extent of any established target organ injury.
- Evaluate possible causes of secondary hypertension.

The following list of investigations would be appropriate in the assessment of diabetic patients with hypertension:

Electrocardiography (ECG)
To determine whether ischaemic heart disease or left ventricular hypertrophy (LVH) is evident. It should be noted that the ECG is not a particularly sensitive method of detecting LVH and an echocardiographic determination of LV mass is preferable when available.

Echocardiography
This investigation is not always widely available to general practitioners but should be. Echocardiography is much more sensitive at detecting LVH and is invaluable for the assessment of patients with evidence of cardiac failure, arrhythmias and murmurs.

Chest X-ray
This investigation is frequently performed, but often provides little additional information when assessing the hypertensive patient. When cardiomegaly is apparent on chest X-ray it is usually evident clinically and certainly obvious by echocardiography.

Urea, creatinine and electrolytes
These are essential to establish whether renal impairment is present and whether there are any electrolyte abnormalities that may point to a diagnosis of secondary hypertension, e.g. hypokalaemia.

Lipoprotein profile
The cholesterol level (LDL and HDL) can be estimated from a non-fasting sample; triglycerides should be estimated from a fasting blood sample.

Glycated haemoglobin A1c
This can give a medium-term index of glycaemic control.

Dipstick urinalysis for blood and protein
If proteinuria is detected, the protein excretion rate should be quantified from a 24-hour urine collection. If the urine is negative for protein on dipstick, the microalbumin excretion rate (or urine albumin:creatinine ratio) should be measured.

Further investigations

Based on the results of the initial investigation, further evaluation may be required, usually within the hospital outpatient setting and usually where a clinical suspicion of secondary hypertension exists:

Renal ultrasound
If renal disease or renal artery stenosis is suspected, a renal ultrasound examination is a useful investigation and preferable to intravenous urography as a first investigation.

Urinary catecholamines and metabolites
This investigation is performed to screen for phaeochromocytoma.

Captopril renogram
This investigation involves the use of radioisotopes to detect a disproportionate decrease in renal function after the administration of a single dose of the ACE inhibitor captopril, in patients with unilateral renal artery stenosis. Other investigations for renovascular disease include the use of real-time colour Doppler and angiography.

Random growth hormone level
Screening for acromegaly where clinical suspicion exists.

24-hour urinary free cortisol
Screening for Cushing's syndrome when clinical suspicion exists.

Plasma renin and aldosterone
Useful when there is a clinical suspicion of secondary hypertension in general and hyperaldosteronism in particular.

REFERENCES

1. Hypertension Detection and Follow-up Program Cooperative Group. Five year findings of the Hypertension Detection and Follow-up Program. I: Reduction in mortality of persons with high blood pressure, including mild hypertension. *JAMA* 1979; **242**: 2562-71.

2. The Systolic Hypertension in the Elderly Program Cooperative Research Group. Implications of the Systolic Hypertension in the Elderly Program. *Hypertension* 1993; **21**: 335-43.

3. The National High Blood Pressure Education Program Working Group. National High Blood Pressure Education Program Working Group report on hypertension in diabetes. *Hypertension* 1994; **23**: 145-58.

4. Sever P, Beevers G, Bulpitt C, Lever A, Ramsay L, Reid J, Swales J. Management guidelines in essential hypertension: report of the second working party of the British Hypertension Society. *Br Med J* 1993; **306**: 983-7.

CHAPTER 6 - SUMMARY POINTS

- A persistently elevated blood pressure of >140/90 mmHg warrants treatment in IDDM patients.
- A persistently elevated blood pressure of >160/90 mmHg warrants treatment in NIDDM patients.
- A blood pressure of >140/90 but <160/90 mmHg requires non-pharmacological intervention in NIDDM patients.
- The treated blood pressure goal is <140/90 in IDDM and <160/90 in NIDDM patients.
- Consider secondary causes (including some drug therapies) of hypertension in diabetic subjects.
- Do not treat blood pressure on the basis of a single reading.

Chapter Seven

THE TREATMENT OF HYPERTENSION IN DIABETIC PATIENTS

Goals of therapy

It is useful to recall the objectives when treating hypertension in diabetic subjects. The main objectives are to delay or prevent the development of macrovascular disease complications such as stroke, myocardial infarction, peripheral vascular disease and heart failure. The effective treatment of hypertension may also delay or prevent the development of microvascular complications, such as nephropathy and possibly also retinopathy and neuropathy.

Antihypertensive therapy: treatment goals

1. To reduce cardiovascular morbidity and mortality

2. To delay or prevent the development of:

- Stroke
- Myocardial infarction
- Left ventricular hypertrophy
- Heart failure
- Peripheral vascular disease
- Diabetic nephropathy
- Retinopathy

Non-pharmacological treatment of hypertension in diabetic subjects

All national guidelines recommend the use of non-pharmacological strategies in the management of hypertension. Non-pharmacological treatment is particularly important in diabetic subjects as environmental and lifestyle factors may be a major determinant of the high prevalence of hypertension in this condition. It is also important to note that non-pharmacological management may not only lower blood pressure, but also reduce the overall CV risk burden of diabetic subjects with hypertension.

The rationale for advocating non-pharmacological intervention is particularly strong for patients with diabetes. In this population such a strategy may assist in reducing blood pressure in those patients with established hypertension and may obviate the need for drug therapy in a significant proportion of patients with mild hypertension. It may minimise the drug requirements for those who require drug treatment. In addition, non-pharmacological treatment may also reduce the risk of cardiovascular disease independent of any change in blood pressure by its favourable effects on insulin sensitivity, dyslipidaemia and glycaemic control. Thus non-pharmacological measures play an important role in any blood pressure management programme and should be offered to all hypertensive patients whether or not they are receiving anti-hypertensive medication.

Non-pharmacological treatment of hypertension

- Reduce energy intake and achieve ideal body weight.
- Reduce saturated fat intake.
- Take regular exercise.
- Stop smoking.
- Avoid excess alcohol intake.
- Reduce salt intake.

Reduction of calorie and fat intake

A majority of hypertensive diabetic subjects are overweight and carry excess fat. There is an overwhelming body of clinical evidence demonstrating that weight reduction can lower blood pressure and improve insulin sensitivity and the associated CV risk-factor profile. Patients should be advised to reduce their total energy intake and to reduce their saturated fat intake. The current dietary recommendations for patients with diabetes, including those with hypertension, are that 50-60% of total energy intake should be via carbohydrates, preferably unrefined carbohydrate. Fat intake should account for less than 30% of total calorie intake. The fibre content of the diet should be doubled.

Restriction of salt intake

Moderate salt restriction has been shown to lower blood pressure in diabetic patients. Diabetic subjects are known to have increased exchangeable total body sodium, and sodium has been implicated in the pathogenesis of hypertension in IDDM and NIDDM (see Chapter 2). Moderate sodium restriction can usually be achieved by eliminating the use of table salt, reducing the use of salt when preparing food and avoiding excessively salty foods. More drastic reductions in salt intake are unlikely to be sustained. These measures, when incorporated into a weight-reducing diet, have been shown to be very impressive at reducing blood pressure, particularly systolic blood pressure.

Avoidance of excess alcohol intake

Chronic excessive alcohol intake is associated with blood pressure elevation. Alcohol intake should be moderated in those with a heavy intake. Women should consume a maximum of 21 units of alcohol per week and men a maximum of 28 units of alcohol per week. It is also important that there are significant numbers of alcohol-free days and that binge drinking is avoided.

Cessation of smoking

Despite the obvious health risks, particularly in those already predisposed to CV disease, many diabetic subjects continue to smoke. Stopping smoking will not reduce blood pressure but it will reduce CV risk. For hypertensive diabetic patients who smoke, cessation of smoking remains a top priority. There is unequivocal evidence that smoking results in a two- to five-fold increase in risk of coronary death and ischaemic stroke in hypertensive patients.

Regular physical exercise

Increasing physical activity modestly reduces blood pressure. However, increased levels of physical activity will often assist in weight reduction programmes and thus become a key part in non-pharmacological management. The term 'exercise' encompasses a wide spectrum of physical activity. There is no doubt that sustained low-level exercise working to a capacity of 40-70% of maximum is more effective at weight reduction and improving aerobic fitness than short bursts of heavy tonic exercise, e.g. weightlifting. An ideal exercise regime would comprise a period of sustained physical activity lasting approximately 30 minutes at least three times per week. In the more physically able and active, this could involve jogging, cycling or swimming etc., or a brisk 30-minute walk three times a week for the less physically able. Such levels of exercise will:

- increase the overall well-being of patients,

- have a modest blood pressure lowering effect,

- facilitate weight reduction, and

- improve insulin sensitivity and the associated dyslipidaemia.

Who will benefit from non-pharmacological treatment?

The simple answer is everybody! This treatment may be sufficient to lower the blood pressure of patients with diabetes with minimal elevations of blood pressure to the normal range. In patients with evidence of target organ injury, drug therapy is added to non-pharmacological treatment to lower blood pressure. While the benefits of non-pharmacological intervention should not be underestimated, there is little doubt that the successful implementation of non-pharmacological strategies to lower blood pressure and reduce CV risk is time consuming and requires considerable effort on the part of the practice nurse and preferably also a dietitian. In the context of providing dietary advice it is also desirable to include other family members in the discussion and continuously to reinforce the importance of this therapeutic approach to the patient. This latter point is particularly important once drug therapy has commenced. Drug therapy does not replace non-pharmacological treatment, the two forms of treatment are complementary.

Summary of non-pharmacological treatment

In diabetic subjects with hypertension, non-pharmacological treatment should be vigorously pursued. In some patients this approach alone may be sufficient to restore blood pressure to the normal range. Where it is not, or when target organ damage already exists, it is an important adjunctive therapy to help lower blood pressure and reduce overall CV risk.

Pharmacological treatment of hypertension in diabetic subjects

Drug therapy is invariably required to treat hypertension adequately in a majority of diabetic subjects. Mindful of the fact that the objectives of treatment are to minimise the overall CV risk burden, the ideal antihypertensive regimen should provide effective control of blood pressure, but must not worsen co-existing CV risk factors. To achieve stable and prolonged blood pressure control, good compliance with therapy is essential and this is more likely to be achieved by drugs that can be administered once daily and have an acceptable side-effect profile. The latter point has particular relevance to diabetic patients whose propensity to orthostatic hypotension, impotence and hypoglycaemia may be adversely influenced by some classes of drug therapy. Moreover, the presence of disease complications, such as peripheral vascular disease, ischaemic heart disease, renal disease and autonomic neuropathy, may all influence the selection of drug therapy for individual patients.

Ideal drug therapy for hypertension in diabetic subjects

- Effective and smooth 24-hour control of blood pressure.

- Does not worsen other cardiovascular risk factors, e.g. lipid profiles.

- Does not adversely influence glycaemic control.

- Once-daily administration.

- Low side-effect profile.

There are five classes of drugs that are routinely used for the management of hypertension, these are:

1. thiazide diuretics,

2. beta-blockers,

3. alpha-blockers,

4. calcium antagonists,

5. ACE inhibitors.

I will review the relative merits and disadvantages of each drug class when considering their use in the management of hypertension in diabetic subjects. The side-effects and adverse effects listed are only those which are of specific relevance to the management of hypertension and its complications in diabetic subjects. For a full account of the recognised side-effects and contraindications to therapy for each class of drug, the reader is referred to the specific drug data sheets.

THIAZIDE DIURETICS

Mode of action

Thiazides (e.g. bendrofluazide) and thiazide-like drugs (e.g. chlorthalidone) act on the luminal aspect of the distal convoluted tubule of the kidney and inhibit the reabsorption of sodium. As this segment of the renal tubule is responsible for only 10% of total renal sodium reabsorption the thiazide diuretics have only a modest natriuretic effect when compared with the loop diuretics. The increased delivery of sodium to the distal tubule promotes sodium:potassium exchange which causes a sustained increase in the renal clearance of potassium, resulting in hypokalaemia. Thiazides also promote the excretion of magnesium and reduce the excretion of calcium and uric acid.

In the acute phase of thiazide therapy, blood pressure is reduced due to volume depletion and a reduced cardiac output which is partially compensated for by an increase in peripheral resistance. With chronic therapy, this acute response is further compensated for by various neurohumoral mechanisms which leads to a new steady state characterised by a minimal reduction in plasma and extracellular fluid volume, a reduction in total peripheral resistance and lower blood pressure.

The hypotensive effect of thiazide diuretics is most pronounced in patients with low plasma renin values, i.e. elderly and Afro-Caribbean hypertensive subjects. It is important to note that the blood pressure response to thiazide diuretics is very flat and dissociated from the dose effect of thiazides on potassium, glucose and lipid profiles. For bendrofluazide, 2.5 mg once daily appears to be the optimal dose to achieve a maximal antihypertensive effect and minimise the metabolic side-effects. For a vast majority of patients, thiazides at higher doses (i.e. bendrofluazide 5 mg and 10 mg daily) will not improve blood pressure control, but will greatly increase the adverse metabolic effects.

Benefits of thiazide therapy

Thiazide diuretics are cheap, tried, tested, reasonably well tolerated and frequently used for the treatment of hypertension. In non-diabetic hypertensive patients, thiazides have been shown to lower blood pressure very effectively and reduce CV morbidity and mortality. Sodium retention is important in the pathogenesis of hypertension in diabetic subjects, thus the natriuretic properties of thiazides would seem to be a logical therapeutic approach. Nevertheless, the use of thiazides in diabetic subjects is in decline. This relates to a number of possible adverse effects which are particularly relevant to hypertensive patients with diabetes.

Potential adverse effects of thiazide diuretics in diabetic subjects with hypertension

Effects of glucose homeostasis
Thiazide diuretics adversely affect carbohydrate metabolism in a dose-dependent manner although these effects are less common with the lower doses now recommended for the management of hypertension. The mechanism for glucose intolerance is unknown but may be related to hypokalaemia. Some studies have suggested that the thiazide-induced glucose intolerance can be diminished by concurrent administration of potassium supplements and the subsequent correction of potassium depletion. There is no doubt that the adverse effects of thiazides on glucose tolerance are further exacerbated when they are co-administered with beta-blockers.

Dyslipidaemia
The capacity of thiazides to increase blood cholesterol levels has been recognised for decades. In addition to promoting an increase in LDL cholesterol, they can reduce HDL cholesterol. Short-term studies in patients treated with thiazides, albeit often in larger doses, have revealed an increase in total cholesterol of approximately 6.5%, a 15% increase in LDL cholesterol, a 23% increase in total triglycerides and a 28% increase in VLDL cholesterol. However, longer-term trials have shown no increase in total cholesterol suggesting that the lipid changes observed in short-term studies were transitory. The adverse effects of thiazides on lipid profiles are certainly potentiated by beta-blockers.

Diabetic complications
Impotence is a significant and vastly under-reported problem in men with diabetes. Thiazides, even at lower doses, have been implicated in the development of impotence. The capacity of thiazides to precipitate, or worsen, impotence becomes an important consideration for males with diabetes who are already at greatly increased risk from this problem.

Sudden cardiac death
Previous reports from prospective clinical trials have suggested that higher-dose thiazide therapy may be associated with an increase in sudden cardiac death in hypertensive patients with pre-existing ECG abnormalities. A more

recent study demonstrated that primary cardiac arrest in hypertensive patients treated with thiazides (diabetic and non-diabetic) was higher in patients receiving higher-dose thiazides and that this risk could be reduced by combining the thiazide with a potassium-sparing diuretic, but not by potassium supplements.

Indapamide
Indapamide is a derivative of thiazide-type diuretics that is as effective as thiazides diuretics at lowering blood pressure in non-diabetic and diabetic subjects. This agent is reported to have a lesser effect on the metabolic profile of diabetic patients. A survey of all the reported data suggests that indapamide (2.5 mg daily) produces a significantly lesser increase in total cholesterol (1.4% increase) when compared to low-dose thiazide therapy (3.8% increase, $p < 0.05$) and also a significantly lesser increase in triglycerides (indapamide 0.5% increase versus low-dose thiazides 10.8% increase, $p < 0.01$). The blood pressure lowering effect of indapamide and low-dose thiazides were equivalent. There is no information about the impact of indapamide on impotence. Moreover, there are no trials demonstrating that indapamide is as effective as thiazides in reducing cardiovascular mortality. Nevertheless, if one of the objectives of antihypertensive therapy is to lower blood pressure without adversely influencing the metabolic profile of diabetic patients, then indapamide may be preferable to standard thiazide therapy when a thiazide is to be added to the antihypertensive regimen of patients with diabetes.

Conclusion
Although thiazides are still widely used as first-line therapy for the management of hypertension in non-diabetic subjects, their adverse effects on glucose tolerance, plasma lipids and potassium, and their capacity to increase the risk of impotence, suggest that these drugs are unsuitable as first-line therapy for a majority of diabetic patients with hypertension. They remain useful agents to potentiate the antihypertensive effect of ACE inhibitors and other agents, and are well-tolerated and very effective for the management of isolated systolic hypertension in the elderly diabetic patient.

BETA-ADRENERGIC BLOCKERS

Mode of action
Beta-blockers inhibit beta-adrenergic receptors and thereby reduce cardiac output, heart rate and renal blood flow. Although peripheral vascular resistance rises, the net effect of all of the haemodynamic changes is a fall in blood pressure. Beta-blockers also decrease plasma renin activity. Beta-blockers also have an anti-arrhythmic action which may be important in

patients with co-existent ischaemic heart disease. They are less effective at lowering blood pressure in 'low renin hypertension', i.e. Afro-Caribbean and elderly patients.

Benefits of beta-blocker therapy

These drugs have been, and are still, widely used in the treatment of hypertension. Like the thiazides, the beta-blockers have been extensively tried and tested in prospective randomised clinical trials, predominantly in nondiabetic hypertensive subjects, and have been shown to reduce CV mortality. Beta-blockers are also important in the management of ischaemic heart disease. They are often very effective in reducing the symptoms of angina and the beneficial effects of long-term beta-blockade following acute myocardial infarction are well documented and must be due, at least in part, to a reduction in death from ventricular tachyarrhythmias.

Potential adverse effects of beta-blocker therapy in diabetic subjects with hypertension

Glucose homeostasis

The perception of symptoms of hypoglycaemia may be impaired or altered by non-selective beta-blockade. This has perhaps been over-emphasised and is much less of a problem if the cardioselective agents are used.

Serum lipids

Both selective and non-selective beta-blockers increase triglycerides and have a potent effect to lower HDL cholesterol. The seemingly small changes in HDL cholesterol may be important as there appears to be a 5.5% reduction in coronary events for every 1 mg/dl increment in HDL cholesterol. Beta-blockers with intrinsic sympathomimetic activity (ISA) tend not to affect lipids so adversely, but in my experience are less effective at lowering blood pressure. Moreover, it cannot be assumed that beta-blockers with ISA afford the same protection following myocardial infarction.

Diabetic complications

Beta-blockers can cause a significant deterioration in peripheral vascular disease due to their action in increasing peripheral vascular resistance. Beta-blockers may also cause significant symptomatic deterioration in patients with left ventricular dysfunction. Beta-blockers may also contribute to impotence. Their effect in this regard is less potent than that seen with thiazide diuretics; nevertheless, these drugs are often combined with thiazide diuretics which may greatly exacerbate the effect on impotence. Beta-blockers also reduce physical activity and have been shown to promote weight gain more readily than other antihypertensive agents. This is another distinct disadvantage when one considers the importance of exercise and weight reduction in the non-pharmacological management of hypertension and CV risk.

Conclusions

These drugs are often effective in lowering blood pressure and are useful in the management of ischaemic heart disease in patients who can tolerate them. Beta-blockers do make the management of diabetes more difficult, they may adversely affect plasma lipids and have an adverse effect on some of the complications of diabetes. Like the thiazides, beta-blockers can also exacerbate insulin resistance and the combination of these agents greatly enhances this effect. Indeed, the dyslipidaemia associated with beta-blocker therapy (increased triglycerides and low HDL-cholesterol) is identical to that observed in insulin resistant individuals. If these drugs are to be used, then a relatively selective beta-blocker is preferred. Nevertheless, with the emergence of newer, metabolically neutral and better-tolerated agents, the use of beta-blockers in the primary management of hypertension in diabetic subjects will continue to decline.

ALPHA$_1$-ADRENERGIC BLOCKERS

Mode of action

Increased activity of the sympathetic nervous system plays a role in the development of increased peripheral vascular resistance, and thus hypertension, in diabetic subjects (see Chapter 2). The peripheral alpha$_1$-adrenergic receptor blockers selectively inhibit post-junctional alpha$_1$-adrenergic receptors with high affinity for the alpha$_1$ receptor. The inhibition of the alpha$_1$ receptor results in vasodilatation and thus reversal of one of the fundamental haemodynamic abnormalities sustaining the elevation of blood pressure in diabetic subjects.

The original drug in this class was prazosin. This was widely used but required two to three daily doses and, with time, tachyphylaxis to its antihypertensive action developed. In my view, there is no indication to continue the use of prazosin to treat hypertension since the development of new longer-acting alpha$_1$-adrenergic blockers such as doxazosin or terazosin.

Doxazosin or terazosin can be administered once daily and both provide excellent 24-hour blood pressure control. Moreover, the problem of tachyphylaxis, which compromised the use of prazosin, does not occur with these newer, longer-acting agents.

Benefits of alpha$_1$-adrenergic blockers

Alpha$_1$-blockers effectively lower blood pressure in patients with and without diabetes. In addition to the benefit of once-daily dosing, there is no absolute contraindication to their use for the management of hypertension. Indeed, there are potential benefits when using alpha-blockers for the management of hypertension in patients with diabetes, particularly those with NIDDM.

Improved insulin sensitivity
The hallmark of NIDDM is the development of insulin resistance, which plays an important role in the development of the associated dyslipidaemia and other metabolic complications (see Chapter 4). Alpha-blocker therapy has been shown to improve insulin sensitivity in NIDDM patients. Thus, as well as treating hypertension, this class of drug specifically targets one of the fundamental metabolic disturbances that contributes to the increased cardiovascular risk associated with diabetes mellitus.

Desirable effects on dyslipidaemia
The ability of alpha-blockers to impact favourably on insulin sensitivity, and thereby reduce insulin resistance, has been shown to improve the dyslipidaemia associated with NIDDM. Typically, insulin resistance is associated with increased circulating triglycerides and decreased HDL cholesterol. Alpha-blocker therapy has been shown to lower total cholesterol, increase HDL cholesterol and lower triglycerides. This action of alpha-blockers is in direct contrast to the worsening of NIDDM-associated dyslipidaemia observed with high-dose thiazide and/or beta-blocker therapy. It is also more impressive than the effects on dyslipidaemia observed with other metabolically neutral drugs, such as ACE inhibitors, calcium channel blockers or angiotensin-II receptor antagonists. These favourable and desirable metabolic actions of alpha-blockers suggest that alpha-blockers are ideally suited to the management of hypertension in patients with diabetes mellitus, particularly NIDDM.

Impotence
Impotence is a significant problem in men with diabetes, and invariably worse following blood pressure lowering with any antihypertensive therapy. The results of the TOMHS (Treatment of Mild Hypertension Study) suggested that impotence was less likely to be induced by alpha-blockers when compared with other therapies, particularly thiazides and beta-blockers.

Prostatic outflow obstruction
Prostatic outflow obstruction is, of course, no more common in men with diabetes than in the non-diabetic male population. Nevertheless, when it does occur, alpha-blockers have a beneficial effect on the symptoms and are widely used by urologists for the management of early prostatic disease. For this reason, alpha-blockers may be a preferred therapy in hypertensive subjects with coincidental prostatic outflow obstruction.

Potential adverse effects of alpha₁-adrenergic blockers in diabetic subjects with hypertension

The best known side-effect of alpha-blockers is their 'first-dose hypotensive effect' culminating in symptomatic orthostatic hypotension in some patients. This is less of a problem with the newer longer-acting alpha-blockers, such as doxazosin and terazosin, but is relevant to the diabetic population in whom clinical or subclinical autonomic neuropathy may render them very susceptible to postural hypotension which can persist beyond the first dose. First-dose hypotension can occur in any patient, but is more likely to occur when alpha-blockers are added to diuretic therapy or in combination with a low-salt diet. These agents should be started in low dose with avoidance of diuretics for at least two days previously. In addition, the patient can be advised to take the medication at bedtime.

Conclusions

The longer-acting alpha-blockers are effective at lowering blood pressure in diabetic subjects and exhibit potentially favourable effects on glucose homeostasis and lipid metabolism. Whether these seemingly beneficial effects on dyslipidaemia ultimately translate into an improved CV prognosis awaits confirmation in clinical trials. Nevertheless, in a population at such high risk of premature CV disease the aim of any therapy must be to impart benefit and not to exacerbate the existing risk. Providing there is no significant evidence of postural hypotension, these agents are often well tolerated and are increasingly used to manage hypertension in IDDM and particularly NIDDM patients. Furthermore, in Asian patients in whom insulin resistance is so common, the favourable effects of alpha-blockers on the metabolic profile is particularly desirable. Alpha-blockers are often very effective at lowering blood pressure in Afro-Caribbean patients whereas beta-blockers and ACE inhibitors are usually less effective. Moreover, in this latter group of patients, the combination of once-daily alpha-blockers with once-daily calcium channel blocker preparations is very potent and often very effective in patients with high blood pressure resistant to monotherapy.

CALCIUM ANTAGONISTS

Mode of action

The influx of calcium into vascular smooth muscle and cardiac myocytes is a crucial cellular event in the initiation of cell contraction. Calcium enters these cells via L-type calcium channels and these channels can be selectively inhibited by the binding of calcium antagonists to the alpha₁ subunit of the channel, inhibiting calcium influx into the vascular smooth muscle of resistance vessels resulting in vasodilatation of these vessels. The resulting fall in peripheral vascular resistance produces a sustained fall in blood pressure.

Although they are often referred to as a single class of agents, the calcium antagonists belong to three distinct chemical groups. Moreover, this distinction may be clinically important in diabetic subjects. The three chemical groupings are:

1. Dihydropyridines: amlodipine, lacidipine, nifedipine and other '... pines'.

2. Benzothiazepines: diltiazem is the only commonly used member of this group.

3. Phenylalkylamines: verapamil is the only commonly used member of this group.

For practical purposes, they are commonly referred to as two groups: the dihydropyridines and the non-dihydropyridines (diltiazem and verapamil). The different chemical properties of these compounds play an important role in determining the characteristics of calcium channel inhibition and their tissue selectivity. For example, verapamil has potent effects on atrioventricular nodal conduction, whereas some of the dihydropyridines do not.

Benefits of calcium antagonists

These agents are very effective at lowering blood pressure in IDDM and NIDDM subjects with hypertension irrespective of age, sex or racial origin. Most of the newer calcium channel blockers can be administered once daily, have a good safety profile and are reasonably well tolerated. They function as vasodilators and thus should not worsen, and could potentially improve, peripheral vascular disease and impotence.

Calcium antagonists have become established as important agents in the management of symptomatic ischaemic heart disease, i.e. angina. Their effectiveness in the primary prevention of myocardial infarction is undergoing assessment in clinical trials. With regard to secondary prevention, a recent meta-analysis on the use of calcium antagonists post-myocardial infarction has suggested that verapamil and diltiazem may reduce the incidence of non-Q-wave infarction.

Calcium antagonists have been shown to be effective at reducing left ventricular hypertrophy in hypertensive subjects. Whilst a recent pooled analysis of over 100 studies suggests that, per mmHg change in blood pressure, calcium antagonists may have a lesser impact on left ventricular mass than ACE inhibitors[1], this is by no means confirmed and some recent studies suggest that the newer longer-acting calcium antagonists have an equal effect on left ventricular mass.

The role of calcium antagonists in the management of diabetic subjects with proteinuria is emerging as an area of considerable debate and controversy. Some evidence suggests that some of the non-dihydropyridines have a powerful antiproteinuric action in hypertensive diabetic patients. This is discussed in greater detail later in this chapter.

One might have expected some of the shorter-acting calcium antagonists to exacerbate postural hypotension in diabetic subjects, particularly when this is due to autonomic neuropathy. However, this appears not to be much of a problem with calcium antagonists in practice.

Another potentially important advantage of calcium antagonists is that they are metabolically neutral. Unlike thiazides and beta-blockers they do not induce insulin resistance and have no reported adverse effects on the lipid profiles of diabetic subjects. Although insulin secretion is a calcium-dependent process, the potential for calcium antagonists to adversely affect glucose homeostasis in diabetic patients has not been revealed in numerous long-term studies.

Potential adverse effects of calcium antagonists in diabetic subjects with hypertension

The main side-effects of calcium antagonists are related to their vasodilator action. These include activation of the sympathetic nervous system resulting in palpitations, sweating, tremor and headache. This effect is observed most commonly with the shorter-acting dihydropyridines and is much less common with the longer-acting dihydropyridines, such as amlodipine. Oedema is another problem related to vasodilatation; it occurs with short- and longer-acting agents and does not respond to diuretic therapy. All of the vasodilator-related side-effects are less common with the non-dihydropyridines. Although the vasodilator-related side-effects and oedema are not specific to diabetic subjects, they can lead to the inappropriate use of diuretics to treat 'calcium antagonist oedema' which can precipitate postural hypotension.

It is also important to note that some calcium antagonists have a negatively inotropic action on the heart, particularly verapamil and diltiazem, and can worsen pre-existing heart failure. Moreover, verapamil can cause prolonged atrial arrest in patients with pre-existing cardiac conduction abnormalities. These effects are much more pronounced when verapamil is combined with a beta-blocker (not recommended!) and also occur to a lesser extent with diltiazem. It has also been suggested that calcium antagonists can exacerbate gastroparesis in diabetics with autonomic neuropathy. However, the most common gastrointestinal side-effect is constipation which is unique to verapamil due to its action to inhibit intestinal smooth muscle contraction; it occurs in approximately 10% of recipients.

Conclusion

Calcium antagonists are widely used for the management of hypertension in IDDM and NIDDM subjects. They are very effective at lowering mild to severe elevations of blood pressure. Moreover, calcium antagonists are frequently and very effectively combined with other agents when more than one is required. The longer-acting calcium antagonists are reasonably well-tolerated and appear to have no clinically relevant metabolic side-effects. Calcium antagonists are useful in diabetic patients with hypertension and/or angina and will not adversely influence renal function in those with renovascular disease. In hypertensive diabetic subjects with microalbuminuria or proteinuria, non-dihydropyridine calcium antagonists appear to have a greater antiproteinuric effect than the dihydropyridines. That issue aside, calcium antagonists are now regarded by many as an important first-line antihypertensive therapy for diabetic subjects.

ANGIOTENSIN CONVERTING ENZYME (ACE) INHIBITORS

The renin-angiotensin system (RAS) plays an important role in the control of blood pressure, and fluid and electrolyte metabolism. Angiotensin converting enzyme (ACE) converts angiotensin-I (AI) to angiotensin-II (AII). AII is a potent vasoconstrictor and stimulates aldosterone secretion. AII has also been strongly implicated in the regulation of vascular growth and remodelling and myocardial hypertrophy in patients with hypertension. ACE inhibitors lower blood pressure by decreasing elevated systemic vascular resistance, but do not (unlike vasodilators) produce reflex sympathetic activation or alter myocardial conductivity. Moreover, by inhibiting the growth-promoting actions of AII, ACE inhibitors could also prevent, or induce regression of, the structural changes of the left ventricle or the walls of resistance vessels that play a role in the maintenance of hypertension.

ACE inhibitors are not specific for angiotensin converting enzyme and also inhibit the action of various kininases, which prevents the natural breakdown of kinins such as bradykinin. Bradykinin can promote the release of endothelium-derived relaxing factors and thus the local build up of bradykinin may contribute to an improvement in endothelial function in patients with diabetes and thereby contribute to the hypotensive actions of ACE inhibitors. However, this inhibition of kininases in the lung may underlie the development of troublesome cough in some patients (see below).

Benefits of ACE inhibitors

ACE inhibitors are established as important agents for the treatment of hypertension and congestive cardiac failure. A majority of ACE inhibitors can be administered as a single daily dose, they are at least as effective at lowering blood pressure as all the aforementioned agents and they maintain this action without the development of tolerance.

ACE inhibitors do not induce insulin resistance and have no detrimental effects on lipid profiles or glycaemic control in diabetic subjects. Some studies have suggested that ACE inhibitors may actually improve insulin sensitivity but this is a minor effect and, like calcium antagonists, they are best classified as metabolically neutral.

Left ventricular hypertrophy (LVH) is a common feature of hypertension in diabetic subjects (see Chapter 3). The development of LVH is an ominous sign and preventing its development or inducing its regression is highly desirable. A recent overview analysis of published clinical trials has concluded that, for any given fall in blood pressure, ACE inhibitors are more effective at inducing LVH regression than any of the other classes of antihypertensive therapy[2].

Many hypertensive diabetic patients also develop heart failure. There is now considerable evidence to suggest that ACE inhibitors not only improve exercise tolerance and symptoms in patients with mild to moderate heart failure, but they also reduce mortality. Unless contraindicated, ACE inhibitors are now established as the drug of choice in hypertensive patients with evidence of LVH and/or heart failure.

A major cause of death in patients with diabetes is coronary heart disease. Clinical studies indicate a protective role for ACE inhibitors after acute myocardial infarction. These studies have demonstrated that ACE inhibitors can delay the development of left ventricular enlargement and thus improve left ventricular function when commenced as early as 24 hours or one to four weeks post-infarction. Moreover, early introduction (3-16 days post-infarction) and subsequent longer-term ACE inhibition (42 months) was associated with improved survival and reduced morbidity and mortality due to major cardiovascular events in post-

---

Table 20 - Summary of post-MI studies with ACE inhibitors, the results of which demonstrate a reduction in mortality versus placebo.

1. Captopril (SAVE Study) - *N Engl J Med* 1992; 327: 669-77.

2. Ramipril (AIRE Study) - *Lancet* 1993; 342: 821-8.

3. Enalapril (CONSENSUS-II) - *N Engl J Med* 1992; 327: 678-84.

4. Captopril (ISIS-4) - *Lancet* 1995; 345: 669-85.

5. Lisinopril (GISSI-3) - *Lancet* 1994; 342: 1115-122.

6. Zofenopril (SMILE Study) - *N Engl J Med* 1995; 332: 80-5.

Treating hypertension

infarction patients with asymptomatic left ventricular dysfunction (see Table 20).

In addition to the potentially beneficial CV effects of ACE inhibitors, this class of drugs is also important in the management of diabetic subjects with incipient diabetic nephropathy (microalbuminuria) and established diabetic nephropathy (proteinuria). ACE inhibitors have been shown to be more effective than conventional antihypertensive therapies at reducing urinary protein excretion and the rate of loss of renal function in IDDM and NIDDM patients. This important action of ACE inhibitors is discussed in more detail later in this chapter.

Potential adverse effects of ACE inhibitors in diabetic patients with hypertension

ACE inhibitors are well-tolerated in the great majority of diabetic patients, but treatment should be commenced with caution in those receiving diuretics or with co-existing autonomic neuropathy because of the possibility of first-dose hypotension. ACE inhibitors should be commenced in low dose and diuretics should be withdrawn for at least 48 hours prior to the first dose.

ACE inhibition promotes potassium retention by the kidney; this can become significant in patients with renal impairment, i.e. diabetic nephropathy, resulting in hyperkalaemia. Hyperkalaemia is more likely to develop when ACE inhibitors are combined with potassium-sparing diuretics (e.g. amiloride or spironolactone), a combination that should be avoided.

ACE inhibitors can also lead to a profound deterioration in renal function in patients with bilateral renal artery stenosis (which may be more common in NIDDM patients, see Chapter 2) or in patients with advanced chronic renal failure of any aetiology. The development of acute renal impairment in these circumstances is usually reversible, but will go undetected until it is very advanced unless the patient's biochemistry is checked before, and within two weeks of commencing, ACE inhibitor therapy (see later in this chapter).

The development of a dry irritant cough occurs in approximately 15% of patients receiving ACE inhibitors. It is no more common in diabetic than non-diabetic subjects but is more common in women. The cough resolves on discontinuation of ACE inhibitor therapy.

Some ACE inhibitors have been reported to be associated with the development of fetal abnormalities in animals and isolated clinical cases. They should not be administered to women of child-bearing potential. This is an important consideration in younger IDDM patients. Finally, ACE inhibitors do not appear to be a major cause of impotence, although impotence can develop with any antihypertensive agent.

Conclusion

ACE inhibitors have become firmly established as a first-line therapy for the management of hypertension in diabetic subjects. They are strongly indicated in patients with LVH or evidence of heart failure. They are also recommended in hypertensive diabetic subjects with microalbuminuria or proteinuria. The potential nephroprotective role of ACE inhibitors in these circumstances is an exciting development in the management of diabetic nephropathy. However, the enthusiasm for the use of ACE inhibitors as nephroprotective agents must not overshadow the rare, but real, potential of these agents to promote an acute deterioration in renal function, particularly in patients with occult renovascular disease. The expanding role of ACE inhibitor therapy post-myocardial infarction will further increase the exposure of IDDM and NIDDM patients to this class of drug therapy and increase the need for vigilant monitoring of patients' biochemistry.

OTHER ANTIHYPERTENSIVE THERAPIES

There are many other classes of drug therapy that effectively lower blood pressure in hypertensive patients. Some of these other drugs are now rarely used in the management of the hypertensive patient with diabetes, because their side-effect profile renders them less desirable than the aforementioned alternatives. There are also newer classes of drug therapy that may ultimately prove to be very useful in hypertensive diabetic subjects, but with which clinical experience is currently limited.

Sympatholytic agents

The centrally acting alpha$_2$-agonists (clonidine hydrochloride and methyldopa) inhibit central efferent sympathetic activity. They are very effective at lowering blood pressure in diabetic patients, but the high incidence of orthostatic hypotension and impotence associated with their use makes them rather unsuitable for diabetic subjects.

Direct vasodilators

These agents (hydralazine and minoxidil) act directly on vascular (predominantly arteriolar) smooth muscle to lower peripheral vascular resistance and thus blood pressure. They induce a profound reflex sympathetic activation (tachycardia and palpitations) and salt and water retention and are therefore usually combined with a beta-blocker and a diuretic. Hydralazine has been used extensively to treat moderately severe hypertension, usually as a second- or third-line agent. Its use has declined considerably in recent years due to its propensity to cause a lupus reaction in a significant proportion of patients and the more recent availability of safer and better-tolerated agents. The use of minoxidil has always been restricted to those patients with severe hypertension, not readily controlled by combinations of other agents. The use of minoxidil is therefore usually best confined to specialist clinicians experienced in the management of severe hypertension.

Angiotensin-II receptor antagonists

Agents that very specifically inhibit the angiotensin-II type-1 receptor (losartan) have recently entered the clinical arena. This new class of antihypertensive therapy directly inhibits the actions of angiotensin-II by blocking its receptor. As this drug is specific for the angiotensin-II receptor and does not inhibit ACE activity, unlike ACE inhibitors it does not induce coughing. Moreover, because this drug inhibits the action of angiotensin-II, it might be expected to have a similar clinical profile of activity to ACE inhibitors. In this regard, losartan is effective at lowering blood pressure and appears to be metabolically neutral in man. Furthermore, it has been shown to be at least as effective as ACE inhibitors in reducing proteinuria in diabetic animals and at improving cardiac function in animals with heart failure. These promising experimental results await confirmation in large-scale clinical trials in man.

Tables 21 and 22 summarise the metabolic and adverse effects of various antihypertensive therapies.

Table 21 - Potential effects of various antihypertensive therapies on the metabolic and cardiovascular risk profile of diabetic subjects with hypertension.						
	Total cholesterol	Triglyceride	HDL	Glucose tolerance	Insulin sensitivity	Exercise tolerance
Thiazide diuretics*	⇑	⇑⇑	⇓⇓	⇓⇓	⇓⇓	⇔
Beta-blockers†	⇔	⇑⇑⇑	⇓⇓	⇓	⇓	⇓
Alpha-blockers	⇓⇓	⇓⇓	⇑	⇔	⇑	⇔
Calcium channel blockers	⇔	⇔	⇔	⇔	⇑⇔	⇔
ACE inhibitors	⇔	⇔	⇔	⇔	⇑⇔	⇔
*Less of a deleterious effect with lower-dose thiazides †Less of a deleterious effect with 'cardioselective' beta-blockers						

Table 22 - Checklist of known and common or important side-effects of different classes of antihypertensive therapy.

Common side-effects	Diuretic	Beta-blocker	ACE inhibitor	Calcium channel blocker	Alpha-blocker
Headache	-	-	-	+	-
Flushing	-	-	-	+	-
Dyspnoea	-	+	-	-	-
Lethargy	-	+	-	-	-
Impotence	+	+	-	-	-
Cough	-	-	+	-	-
Gout	+	-	-	-	-
Oedema	-	-	-	+	-
Postural hypotension	+	-	+	-	+
Cold hands and feet	-	+	-	-	-

Initiating drug therapy in hypertensive diabetic subjects
In a significant majority of diabetic patients with hypertension, drug therapy will be required to maintain adequate control of blood pressure.

Drug therapy should not be initiated on the basis of a single blood pressure reading; a period of observation is necessary to define the prevailing blood pressure level. The length of this observation period will vary from days to months depending on the severity of the patient's hypertension and whether or not target organ damage is already established. If there is evidence of target organ injury, i.e. left ventricular hypertrophy, proliferative or hypertensive retinopathy, proteinuria, cerebrovascular or ischaemic heart disease, then non-pharmacological treatment alone is unlikely to be sufficient and drug therapy should be initiated to ensure tight blood pressure control. In such patients it is important, however, to continue with lifestyle modifications as they assist in reducing the overall CV risk burden. In patients with less severe elevations of blood pressure, or isolated systolic hypertension and in whom there is no evidence of established target organ injury, a period of observation (three to six months) with the implementation of lifestyle modifications should be tried to determine whether these measures alone reduce blood pressure to the normal range. If not, then drug therapy should be commenced, complemented by continuation of lifestyle modification.

Follow-up of diabetic patients with hypertension
The long-term maintenance of an effective treatment regimen requires regular follow-up. The frequency of follow-up will depend on the characteristics of the individual patient, usually ranging from three- to six-monthly review in patients on antihypertensive medication. At the follow-up visit, the opportunity should also be taken to reinforce the advice about non-pharmacological strategies with continuing encouragement of patients to adopt these important lifestyle changes. In some patients, it is possible to reduce the dose or the number of antihypertensive medications, or indeed withdraw drugs completely. This should not be done without provision for long-term review, and drugs should never be withdrawn in patients with evidence of target organ injury attributed to hypertension.

Drug therapy selection
There are three classes of drug therapy which are increasingly used in diabetic patients as 'first-line agents'; these are the ACE inhibitors, alpha$_1$-blockers and calcium antagonists (Figure 31). The thiazide diuretics in low dose are still useful first-line agents in older diabetic patients with isolated systolic hypertension and to complement the antihypertensive effect of the 'first-line agents' when more than one drug is necessary to control blood pressure. Beta-blockers may also be preferentially used in some patients with angina, after a recent myocardial infarction or to complement the antihypertensive effect of other agents.

One of the major factors dictating the selection of drug therapy will be the presence or absence of specific types of target organ injury, i.e. diabetic nephropathy or the various complications of diabetes that may be favourably or unfavourably influenced by different classes of drugs. Table 23 summarises the various factors that influence the selection of drug therapy.

Combination therapy
In a significant proportion of patients more than one class of drug therapy will be required to gain and maintain adequate blood pressure control. As suggested by the British Hypertension Society, drug combinations to treat hypertension should be based on three principles:

1. Drugs that act at different sites of the blood pressure regulatory mechanism often have complementary actions.

2. The reflex compensatory response to one drug may be counteracted by a second drug.

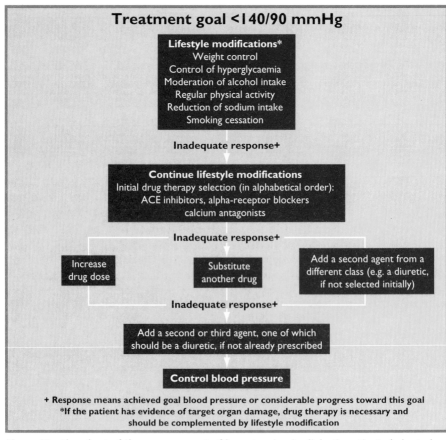

Treatment goal <140/90 mmHg

Lifestyle modifications*
Weight control
Control of hyperglycaemia
Moderation of alcohol intake
Regular physical activity
Reduction of sodium intake
Smoking cessation

Inadequate response+

Continue lifestyle modifications
Initial drug therapy selection (in alphabetical order):
ACE inhibitors, alpha-receptor blockers
calcium antagonists

Inadequate response+

Increase drug dose

Substitute another drug

Add a second agent from a different class (e.g. a diuretic, if not selected initially)

Inadequate response+

Add a second or third agent, one of which should be a diuretic, if not already prescribed

Control blood pressure

+ Response means achieved goal blood pressure or considerable progress toward this goal
*If the patient has evidence of target organ damage, drug therapy is necessary and should be complemented by lifestyle modification

Figure 31 - Flowchart of the management of hypertension in diabetic patients (adapted from current US guidelines specifically designed for diabetic subjects with hypertension [see Chapter 6]).

3. Suboptimal doses of two agents may avoid the side-effects of higher doses of a single drug.

Logical therapeutic combinations

- **ACE inhibitors** + low-dose thiazide diuretics or calcium antagonists.

- **Calcium antagonists** + ACE inhibitor, alpha$_1$-blocker or beta-blocker (not beta-blocker if non-dihydropyridine calcium antagonist).

- **Alpha$_1$-blocker** + calcium antagonist or beta-blocker.

Table 23 - Choice of antihypertensive medication in diabetes with complications.

Complication	Choices	Precautions
Orthostatic hypotension	Calcium antagonists ACE inhibitors Beta-blockers	Methyldopa Alpha-adrenoreceptor blockers
Poor glucose lipid control	Alpha-adrenergic antagonists Calcium antagonists ACE inhibitors	Beta-blockers Diuretics
Hypoglycaemia	None	Beta-blockers
Angina	Calcium antagonists Beta-blockers	None
Post-myocardial infarction	ACE inhibitors Beta-blockers	None
Left ventricular hypertrophy	Alpha-adrenoreceptor blockers Calcium antagonists ACE inhibitors Beta-blockers	Diuretics Direct vasodilators
Peripheral vascular disease	Alpha-adrenoreceptor blockers Calcium antagonists	ACE inhibitors Beta-blockers
Impotence	Alpha-adrenoreceptor blockers Calcium antagonists ACE inhibitors	Methyldopa Clonidine Thiazide diuretics
Microalbuminuria	ACE inhibitors	None
Proteinuria	Non-dihydropyridine calcium antagonists ACE inhibitors	None
Sodium retention (creatinine <200 μmol/l)	Alpha-adrenoreceptor blockers Calcium antagonists ACE inhibitors Thiazide diuretics	None
Sodium retention (creatinine >200 μmol/l)	Loop diuretics	
Hyporeninaemic hypoaldosteronism (hyperkalaemia)	Diuretics	ACE inhibitors Calcium antagonists

DRUG THERAPY SELECTION IN SPECIFIC CLINICAL SITUATIONS

Hypertensive IDDM subjects with no microalbuminuria or proteinuria

IDDM patients most commonly suffer hypertension in association with diabetic nephropathy. In IDDM patients without microalbuminuria or proteinuria, it is likely that the underlying diagnosis is essential hypertension. The choice of first-line agent is between an ACE inhibitor, calcium antagonist or alpha$_1$-blocker. All are effective at lowering blood pressure. If there is evidence of left ventricular hypertrophy an ACE inhibitor may be preferred. However, in females of child-bearing potential, ACE inhibitors in particular should be avoided. If angina is present a calcium antagonist +/- a beta-blocker may be indicated. If the patient has a significant dyslipidaemia then an alpha$_1$-blocker may have a more favourable effect than other agents on the lipid profile. Thiazide diuretics and beta-blockers are much less used as first-line therapy in these patients because of concern over their capacity to influence adversely the patient's metabolic profile and their greater propensity to precipitate impotence.

Hypertensive NIDDM subjects with no microalbuminuria or proteinuria

Non-pharmacological management involving the introduction of lifestyle changes is particularly important in these patients. Many of them are overweight and the associated dyslipidaemia responds to weight reduction and an increase in exercise. Many physicians avoid the use of beta-blockers and thiazides as first-line agents in this group of patients. Thiazides, even in low dose, have the disadvantage of exacerbating the underlying insulin resistance syndrome which is the basis of their disease. This could lead to worsening of pre-existing dyslipidaemia and glucose tolerance. Beta-blockers also share the disadvantage of exacerbating the dyslipidaemia. In particular, they promote a reduction in HDL cholesterol which is already low in many patients with insulin resistance and NIDDM. Beta-blockers also have the disadvantage of reducing the likelihood of an increase in physical activity and thus tend to promote weight gain.

ACE inhibitors, calcium antagonists and alpha$_1$-blockers are increasingly used as first-line agents in NIDDM subjects with hypertension. All are metabolically neutral and thus less likely than thiazide diuretics or beta-blockers to influence adversely the patient's metabolic profile. There has been concern regarding the use of ACE inhibitors in NIDDM patients. This relates to the fact that these patients are usually older and therefore have a higher prevalence of co-existing large vessel atheromatous disease. There is therefore a theoretical risk that these patients will have co-existing renovascular disease (see Chapter 2). While this argument appears logical, in the reality of clinical practice very large numbers of NIDDM patients have been safely established on ACE inhibitor therapy without any deterioration in renal function. Unless there is persuasive clinical evidence for suspecting reno-vascular disease, it is inappropriate to deny a NIDDM patient ACE inhibitor therapy, particularly if there are strong indications, i.e. left ventricular hypertrophy or dysfunction, overt heart failure, the presence of microalbu-minuria or proteinuria, or in patients post-myocardial infarction. Guidance on commencing ACE inhibitor therapy is given later in this chapter in the section dealing with renovascular disease.

Alpha$_1$-selective adrenergic blocking drugs are increasingly used in the management of hypertension associated with NIDDM, although they can cause postural hypotension, particularly in patients with subclinical or overt autonomic neuropathy. An attractive effect of alpha-blockers is their capacity to induce potentially beneficial changes in the dyslipidaemia asso-ciated with NIDDM due to their beneficial effects on insulin sensitivity.

Calcium antagonist are popular first-line agents for the management of hypertension in patients with NIDDM. They have neutral effects on the metabolic syndrome and do not precipitate a decline in renal function in patients with co-existing renovascular disease. Moreover, despite being vasodilators, they are less likely to induce significant postural hypotension even in patients with autonomic neuropathy. They are also useful in patients with co-existing symptomatic angina. For these reasons they are considered to be well-tolerated and effective drugs in the management of hypertension in NIDDM.

In summary, in this category of patient, ACE inhibitors, alpha-blockers and calcium antagonists have become established as first-line agents for the management of hypertension, the final selection depending on the individ-ual patient profile.

Isolated systolic hypertension in diabetic subjects

Many patients with diabetes develop isolated systolic hypertension (ISH) i.e. SBP >160 mmHg associated with a normal DBP <90 mmHg. ISH develops as a consequence of structural changes in the larger blood vessels which leads to a reduction in vascular compliance. As these changes develop as a natural consequence of ageing, ISH is most common in the elderly. Diabetes mellitus accelerates this vascular ageing process, thus ISH is more common and occurs earlier in the ageing diabetic population than in the non-diabet-ic population. Attitudes towards the treatment of ISH have changed marked-ly as a consequence of recent clinical trial data demonstrating the efficacy of antihypertensive therapy in reducing the risk of stroke and ischaemic heart disease mortality in the under-80 age group with ISH. There is no trial data to confirm similar efficacy in younger (age <60 years) subjects with ISH, but by extrapolation it is reasonable to conclude that a similar threshold SBP of 160 mmHg should be considered an indication for treatment in younger patients as well, irrespective of their DBP. Low-dose thiazide diuretics have been shown to be particularly effective in these trials and are recommended as first-line treatment in elderly diabetic subjects with ISH. The treatment goal is to reduce SBP to below 160 mmHg. If a second drug is necessary, ACE inhibitors and/or calcium antagonists are generally efficacious and well-tolerated. ACE inhibitors may also provide additional therapeutic benefits in elderly patients with congestive heart failure. It is emphasised, however, that the measurement of supine and standing blood pressures is particularly important in the management of ISH in elderly patients and severe postural hypotension should be avoided.

Diabetic autonomic neuropathy and supine hypertension with orthostatic hypotension

A significant fall in standing blood pressure (i.e. fall in DBP and/or SBP of >10 mmHg) is observed in approximately 12% of patients with diabetes mellitus, and is more common in the elderly and in those with overt or subclinical autonomic neuropathy. This orthostatic hypotension is frequently associated with supine hypertension and is most difficult to treat. Occasionally the upright blood pressure falls to such an extent that patients are unable to assume an upright posture. This condition is readily aggravated by many antihypertensive medications, particularly the centrally-acting sympatholytic agents (methyldopa and clonidine) and the alpha$_1$-adrenoceptor blockers, and these drugs should be avoided.

To reduce symptoms, the goal of therapy is to increase or maintain the upright pressure and lower the supine pressure. Low-salt diets should be avoided as should diuretic therapy. To increase or maintain the upright pressure, fludrocortisone, which produces sodium retention and can increase blood volume, can be used in small doses of 0.05-0.2 mg daily. However, this medication can further elevate the supine blood pressure and precipitate heart failure. Good elastic hose stockings, personally fitted to cover the legs, perhaps to the waist level, are sometimes beneficial. To lower the supine blood pressure, drugs and mechanical manoeuvres can be employed. Shorter-acting vasodilators, such as ACE inhibitors (e.g. captopril) and/or shorter acting calcium antagonists (e.g. nifedipine), can be taken shortly before bedtime to reduce nocturnal supine blood pressure. The initial dose should be small and slowly titrated upward to prevent orthostatic hypotension in the morning hours. Mechanically elevating the head of the bed 25 cm can also help to allow gravity to decrease supine blood pressure. Close specialist attention and considerable patient encouragement is invariably required to manage this frustrating condition.

Impotence in diabetic subjects with hypertension

Hypertension, neuropathy, vascular insufficiency, psychological problems and also the medication prescribed for hypertension have all been implicated in the development of impotence, impaired ejaculation and decreased libido in men, and decreased vaginal lubrication, orgasmic dysfunction and decreased libido in women. Any antihypertensive medication can contribute to the development of impotence, some more so than others. This should be an important consideration in evaluating patients with both hypertension and diabetes. Thiazides have been implicated in the development of impotence in non-diabetic males and appear to greatly exacerbate the situation in diabetic subjects. Along with thiazides, centrally-acting sympatholytic agents (methyldopa and clonidine) have also gained notoriety with men and their partners. Although impotence can also occur with ACE inhibitors, alpha$_1$-blockers and calcium antagonists, these agents appear to be less troublesome in this respect. It is important to counsel diabetic patients before and after commencing antihypertensive therapy to determine whether impotence may have developed as a consequence of a specific class of treatment. If so, an alternative agent can be tried, but sadly doesn't always straighten things out.

Left ventricular hypertrophy in diabetic subjects with hypertension

For any given level of blood pressure, left ventricular hypertrophy (LVH) appears to be more common in diabetic subjects than those without diabetes (see Chapter 3). LVH is an ominous development and is associated with dramatically increased risk of CHD, sudden cardiac death, congestive cardiac failure and stroke. LVH is thus regarded as one of the most potent indicators of a poor CV prognosis. Recent trials also suggest that antihypertensive therapies that induce regression of LVH are associated with an improved overall prognosis when compared to those therapies which do not. Thus, preventing LVH and/or inducing its regression is a major goal of antihypertensive therapy. Controlling blood pressure with any of the major classes of antihypertensive drugs reduces left ventricular mass, perhaps with the exception of the direct vasodilators. There is also controversy regarding the efficacy of thiazide diuretics with regard to LVH regression. Two recent independent overviews have analysed published clinical trial data on the effects of various antihypertensive drugs on left ventricular structure in hypertensive patients[1,2]. In these meta-analyses, it appeared that, per equivalent reduction in blood pressure, ACE inhibitor therapy induced a greater reduction in left ventricular mass in patients with established LVH than treatment with beta-blockers, calcium antagonists or diuretics. Thus, ACE inhibitors have become a popular first-line therapy in hypertensive patients with LVH.

Left ventricular dysfunction and congestive heart failure in diabetic patients with hypertension

Hypertension is a major cause of congestive cardiac failure. In diabetic subjects with long-standing hypertension, the development of left ventricular dysfunction is particularly common. Whether a specific diabetic cardiomyopathy also contributes to the high incidence of heart failure is still the subject of debate (see Chapter 3). In hypertensive diabetic patients with clinical evidence of left ventricular dysfunction or overt heart failure, first-line antihypertensive therapy is ACE inhibition, usually in combination with a small dose of a loop diuretic (frusemide or bumetanide). This recommendation is supported by clinical trial data demonstrating decreased symptoms and mortality in patients with chronic mild to moderate heart failure (NYHA functional class I - III) and a low ejection fraction when treated with ACE inhibitors. These benefits with ACE inhibition were greater than those observed with the previously more conventional vasodilator therapy (hydralazine and isosorbide dinitrate). The non-dihydropyridine calcium antagonists, in particular verapamil but also diltiazem, can precipitate heart failure in patients with left ventricular dysfunction and should be avoided in patients with poor cardiac function.

Ischaemic heart disease and post-myocardial infarction in diabetic patients with hypertension

Ischaemic heart disease is common in patients with long-standing diabetes and particularly in those with co-existent hypertension. Calcium antagonists and beta-blockers are both useful in the management of patients with a combination of angina and hypertension.

Post-myocardial infarction, both beta-blockers and ACE inhibitors have been shown to improve patient survival. There is also evidence suggesting that non-dihydropyridine calcium antagonists (verapamil and diltiazem) improve survival following a non-Q-wave myocardial infarction. As many patients with ischaemic heart disease are also hypertensive, the aforementioned considerations will influence the prescribing of their medication.

Renal artery stenosis in diabetic subjects with hypertension

The development of renal artery stenosis is, in part, age related and thus more common in patients with NIDDM rather than IDDM. It is also more common in males and smokers. Renovascular disease is not a major cause of hypertension in diabetic subjects but its presence can lead to a decline in renal function in patients prescribed ACE inhibitor therapy. As ACE inhibitor therapy is increasingly used to manage hypertension in diabetic subjects, assessment of patients for possible renal impairment and/or renovascular disease is essential. Renovascular disease is not usually present in patients in whom there is no clinical evidence of vascular disease elsewhere. The absence of foot pulses, and the presence of carotid bruits, femoral bruits, abdominal aortic aneurysm or renovascular bruits must always alert the attention of the physician to the possibility that the hypertension in that particular diabetic patient may be associated with renovascular disease. If a patient has renal bruits, ACE inhibitors should not be prescribed until the patient has undergone further specialist evaluation. The presence of vascular disease elsewhere is not a contraindication, but it does stress the need for special vigilance. Whenever an ACE inhibitor is to be used, it is imperative that renal function is monitored closely. This should involve a check of serum urea, creatinine and potassium prior to the administration of a low dose of ACE inhibitor therapy and a further assessment of renal function, one week after the administration of the test dose. If there has been no disturbance in renal function, the dose of ACE inhibitor can be progressively titrated upward until blood pressure is controlled. Renal function should be checked again after any increase in the dose of ACE inhibitor and certainly a second assessment of renal function should take place within three months of commencing an ACE inhibitor, to ensure that there has been no slowly progressive deterioration in function which can sometimes occur.

If renal function does deteriorate within a week of the test dose, the ACE inhibitor should be stopped and the patient referred for further specialist evaluation. It is conceivable in these circumstances that the patient may have a renovascular stenosis that is amenable to treatment.

In patients with renovascular disease not amenable to corrective treatment, calcium antagonists are the most commonly used first-line agent. However, hypertension can be severe and difficult to treat in these patients who often require a combination of antihypertensive agents.

Ethnic differences in response to antihypertensive therapy
It is well accepted that in patients of Afro-Caribbean origin the antihypertensive effects of beta-blockers and ACE inhibitors are diminished. In these patients, calcium antagonists and alpha$_1$-blockers have proved to be popular and effective first-line alternatives, either alone or in combination.

Diabetic nephropathy, microalbuminuria and proteinuria
Diabetic nephropathy is the single most common cause of end-stage renal disease in the Western world and has already been discussed in some detail in Chapter 5. Microalbuminuria predicts overt nephropathy (proteinuria) and a progressive decline in renal function. Microalbuminuria and proteinuria are also associated with a massive increase in CV morbidity

and mortality (Chapter 5). It has long been recognised that the effective treatment of hypertension with many different types of medication can retard the rate of loss of renal function in patients with diabetic nephropathy. More recent debate has focused on whether the various classes of antihypertensive therapy are equipotent at reducing proteinuria and protecting the kidney. This debate was initially fuelled by studies on diabetic animals which suggested that different classes of antihypertensive therapy have disparate renal protective effects. This important question has been evaluated in numerous clinical trials which have compared the effectiveness of different classes of antihypertensive in reducing urinary albumin excretion. Two recent overview meta-analyses of these various trials reached similar conclusions[3,4], notably that:

1) Despite similar blood pressure reductions, ACE inhibitors were much more effective at reducing urinary protein excretion in diabetic patients than conventional therapy (diuretics or beta-blockers) or calcium antagonists. (There are too few studies at present to draw any specific conclusions about alpha$_1$-blockers.)

2) Unlike other agents, ACE inhibitors appear to exert an antiproteinuric effect even when they do not lower blood pressure.

3) This potentially beneficial effect of ACE inhibitors is a 'class effect' and is not restricted to a specific type of drug formulation (Table 24)[4]. The antiproteinuric effect of ACE inhibitors is impressive.

From the data given in Table 24, it can be deduced that per % reduction in mean systemic blood pressure, ACE inhibitors are associated with a 3.8% reduction in proteinuria compared to a 2.3% reduction in proteinuria per % blood pressure reduction with beta-blockers and diuretics and a 1.5% reduction in proteinuria with calcium antagonists. It is noteworthy, however, that as much as 25% of the antiproteinuric actions of ACE inhibitors occurs at zero blood pressure change, whereas for other agents reduced protein excretion is only apparent when blood pressure is reduced. This distinction has important therapeutic implications for the management of microalbuminuria and proteinuria in normotensive diabetic subjects (see below).

Another intriguing observation from this meta-analysis is that there may be marked differences in the antiproteinuric potency of dihydropyridine and non-dihydropyridine calcium antagonists.

Calcium antagonists in hypertensive diabetic subjects with microalbuminuria and proteinuria
The results of several studies have suggested that dihydropyridine (mostly short-acting) calcium antagonists (nifedipine being the most commonly

Type of therapy	N		Mean study duration (mo)	Average changes (%)	
	Reports	Subjects		Mean systemic BP	Urinary albumin or protein
Diuretics and/or β-blockers	21	258	15.5 (9/22)	-10 (-12/-8)	-23 (-35/-11)
ACE inhibitors	68	1061	8.2 (6/11)	-12 (-19/-5)	-45 (-64/-25)
Ca²⁺ antagonists					
all	27	398	5.4 (3/7)	-12 (-15/-10)	-17 (-33/-2)
nifedipine	12	166	5.9 (3/9)	-13 (-17/-9)	+5 (-21/+31)
all except nifepidine	15	232	5.0 (2/8)	-11 (-14/-7)	-35 (-47/-24)

Mean (95% confidence interval)
*p <0.05

Table 24 - Antiproteinuric action of antihypertensive drugs in diabetics: meta-analysis.

studied) are less effective at reducing proteinuria in hypertensive diabetic animals and man than the non-dihydropyridines (verapamil and diltiazem). This difference in efficacy is thought to relate, in part, to subtle differences in the actions of these two classes of calcium antagonist on renal haemodynamics. While the antiproteinuric effect of non-dihydropyridine calcium antagonists in numerical terms approaches that of ACE inhibition, the antiproteinuric actions of the dihydropyridines have been less impressive despite equivalent reductions in blood pressure (Table 24). The clinical significance of these differential effects is not yet clear, but if a prime objective of therapy is not only to reduce blood pressure, but also to reduce or limit the rise in proteinuria, then it would be prudent to select a non-dihydropyridine calcium antagonist before a short-acting dihydropyridine when treating hypertension in diabetic subjects with microalbuminuria or proteinuria. At present, this distinction is not relevant to hypertensive diabetic subjects without microalbuminuria or proteinuria.

Is it important to lower urinary protein excretion in diabetic subjects?

The observation that an increased urinary albumin excretion rate is associated with a greatly increased likelihood that the diabetic subject will develop renal, microvascular and CV disease has led to the assumption that therapeutic manoeuvres that reduce the albumin excretion rate must be particularly beneficial. This seemingly logical conclusion appears to be true, at least in terms of renal protection. A number of clinical studies have now confirmed that drug-induced reductions in urinary protein excretion in diabetic subjects are associated with greater renal protection than therapies which are less effective at reducing proteinuria; an example from a study in NIDDM patients is shown in Figure 32[5]. Moreover, a large prospective study of ACE inhibitor therapy by Lewis *et al* (see Table 25) confirmed the beneficial effects of reducing proteinuria in IDDM patients in terms of slowing the progression of renal disease and reducing overall mortality[6]. The table shows the outcome events of patients receiving an ACE inhibitor (captopril) during a median follow-up of three years. There was approximately a 50% reduction in events in those receiving the ACE inhibitor.

In conclusion, in patients with an increased urinary albumin excretion rate, a therapy-induced reduction in proteinuria is very desirable, is usually indicative of a reduction in renal injury and may also be associated with an improved overall prognosis.

IDDM patients with hypertension and microalbuminuria or proteinuria
The importance of effective control of blood pressure in these patients cannot be overstated. The goal of treatment must be to maintain the blood pressure below 140/90 mmHg. Others have suggested that even more aggressive targets might be appropriate, e.g. 130/85 mmHg, if such a pressure can be achieved and tolerated. As these patients are also at grave risk from CV disease, it is important that their metabolic control is optimised and other CV risk factors are addressed, e.g. dyslipidaemia. Most physicians would use an ACE inhibitor as first-line antihypertensive therapy in these patients. This choice has been prompted by many clinical studies demonstrating a greater effect of ACE inhibitors than other agents at reducing proteinuria in IDDM patients[3,4]. This impression was substantially supported by the results of a large randomised clinical trial reported by Lewis *et al* in 1993 (Table 25)[6]. In this study, IDDM patients with proteinuria (>0.5 g/day) and early evidence of renal impairment (creatinine <220 μmol/l) were randomised to receive an ACE inhibitor (captopril 25 mg tds) or placebo for a median follow-up of three years. Two hundred and seven patients received captopril, and 202 placebo, in addition to any existing antihypertensive medication they were receiving. Fifty nine per cent of patients in the placebo group and 60% of patients in the ACE inhibitor group were receiving antihypertensive medication at the start of the study. The goal of therapy was to maintain the patients' blood pressure below 140/90 mmHg. This

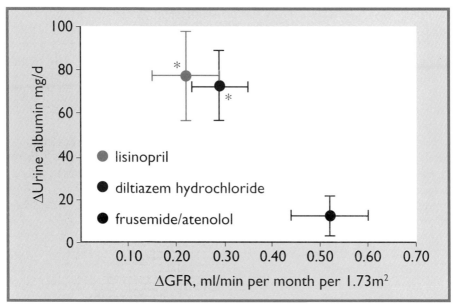

Figure 32 - The average monthly reduction in albuminuria and rate of decline in glomerular filtration rate (GFR) after 18 months of antihypertensive therapy with one of three different classes of agents. An inverse relationship was seen between the amount of renal function preservation and the amount of decline in albuminuria. An asterisk indicates p<0.05, significantly different from frusemide/atenolol with regard to rate of reduction in GFR or proteinuria.

Table 25 - The effect of ACE inhibition in IDDM subjects with diabetic nephropathy.			
	Captopril (207)	Placebo (202)	
Event	Number of patients		p value
Death	8	14	<0.01
Dialysis/ transplantation	20	31	<0.01
Doubling of serum creatinine	25	43	0.007
409 patients randomised Median follow-up: three years (range: 1.8 - 4.8) Mean arterial BP: captopril: 96 ± 8 vs. placebo 100 ± 8 mmHg			

was very effectively achieved and, at most times, the differences in blood pressure between the two groups did not exceed 2 mmHg. Despite statistically similar blood pressure control between the groups, ACE inhibitor therapy was associated with a 50% reduction in the risk of combined end-points (Table 25). This important study corroborated previous data suggesting that ACE inhibitor therapy can improve the renal prognosis of IDDM patients with proteinuria via mechanisms which are not solely dependent on blood pressure reduction.

Monotherapy with ACE inhibitors is rarely sufficient to provide adequate blood pressure control in diabetic patients with proteinuria. In such circumstances, a low-dose thiazide diuretic and/or non-dihydropyridine calcium antagonist can be added to the therapy. The ACE inhibitor/calcium antagonist combination is particularly potent and free of metabolic complications, and is thus likely to become established as the favoured therapy. If an ACE inhibitor is contraindicated or ineffective (i.e. Afro-Caribbean), a non-dihydropyridine calcium antagonist would be a logical first choice.

In patients with established renal impairment, a syndrome of hyporeninaemic hypoaldosteronism commonly develops which predisposes to hyperkalaemia. For this reason potassium-sparing diuretics (e.g. amiloride or spironolactone) should be avoided. The hyperkalaemia can also be exacerbated by the potassium-sparing actions of ACE inhibition.

Salt and water retention is a common early development in patients with renal impairment and may contribute very significantly to the blood pressure elevation. It is very difficult to control the blood pressure of these patients without a diuretic agent, especially when the renal function is significantly impaired. If the serum creatinine is <200 μmol/l, a thiazide diuretic or low-dose loop diuretic (e.g. frusemide 20-40 mg/day) will usually be adequate. If the renal function is more significantly impaired, serum creatinine >200 μmol/l, then much larger doses of loop diuretic will be required to ensure an adequate diuresis (e.g. frusemide 80-250 mg daily). The use of diuretics also helps prevent hyperkalaemia developing.

In conclusion, ACE inhibitors are recommended as first-line therapy in hypertensive IDDM patients with microalbuminuria or proteinuria. If more than one agent is required to control blood pressure, an ACE inhibitor should form part of the therapeutic regimen unless contraindicated. Whatever treatment is adopted, the overriding priority is to control blood pressure.

NIDDM patients with hypertension and microalbuminuria and proteinuria

Microalbuminuria and proteinuria are equally ominous developments in NIDDM patients in whom they are also predictive of renal disease, but more powerfully predict a premature CV death. There are fewer studies comparing the effects of antihypertensive therapy on proteinuria in NIDDM patients. Nevertheless, those studies which have been reported have reached similar conclusions to those in IDDM patients, i.e. that ACE inhibitors have a greater antiproteinuric effect than other agents,[7,8] and that the non-dihydropyridine calcium antagonists are more effective than the dihydropyridines at reducing proteinuria. It has also been demonstrated that the greater the antiproteinuric action of antihypertensive therapy in NIDDM patients, the greater the preservation of renal function (see Figure 33). Importantly, whether drugs with a more powerful antiproteinuric action also improve the CV prognosis (the major cause of premature

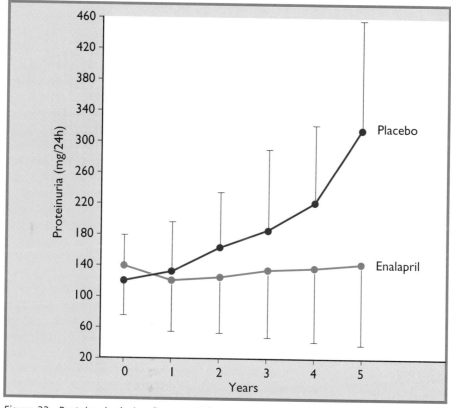

Figure 33 - Proteinuria during five-year follow-up in normotensive NIDDM subjects treated with enalapril (10 mg od) or placebo. Each point represents an annual average of three to four determinations per patient per year. Less proteinuria occurred in the ACE inhibitor group versus placebo after the second year: p <0.05 for second year; p <0.01 for third year; p <0.005 for fourth and fifth years.

death) of NIDDM patients with proteinuria and microalbuminuria, awaits confirmation.

In conclusion, the prescribing strategy for hypertensive NIDDM patients with microalbuminuria and proteinuria should follow that suggested above for IDDM patients. It is likely, however, that a slightly greater proportion of NIDDM patients may be unsuitable for ACE inhibition due to a higher frequency of renovascular disease.

Normotensive IDDM patients with microalbuminuria

It has been suggested that because microalbuminuria is a powerful surrogate marker of ongoing vascular and renal injury, then diabetic patients with an elevated albumin excretion rate may benefit from therapeutic manoeuvres that lower their albumin excretion rate, irrespective of whether or not they are hypertensive. The definition of hypertension is, after all, an arbitrary one. Moreover, it has become abundantly clear that subtle abnormalities in blood pressure regulation have already developed in diabetic subjects with microalbuminuria (see Chapter 5), raising the question as to whether the concept of a normotensive microalbuminuric diabetic subject is in fact a misnomer. There is now increasing evidence to suggest that normotensive IDDM patients with persistent microalbuminuria will benefit from treatment with ACE inhibitor therapy.

The use of ACE inhibitors in these circumstances does not usually produce a marked fall in blood pressure, but does often reduce the urinary albumin excretion rate towards the normal range or at least prevent its otherwise inexorable rise. In a recent European multicentre study[9], 92 patients with persistent microalbuminuria, but no hypertension, were randomised to receive either an ACE inhibitor (captopril) or placebo. After two years, 30% of those allocated to placebo had progressed to nephropathy whereas only 10% receiving the ACE inhibitor had done so. This represents a 60% reduction in risk of progressing to overt nephropathy. This and other studies support the conclusion that ACE inhibitor therapy is beneficial at retarding the progression of renal disease in normotensive IDDM patients. Whether this effect is specific for ACE inhibition or relates to the often small, but significant, falls in blood pressure that tend to occur when normotensive patients are treated awaits further study.

In conclusion, the stakes are high and the odds are stacked against normotensive IDDM patients with persistent microalbuminuria. The current evidence suggests that these patients would benefit from ACE inhibitor therapy. A more cautious approach would be to treat only those patients with evidence of a progressive rise in urinary albumin excretion. The preferred dose of ACE inhibitor in these circumstances is unclear. Empirically, captopril was administered at 50 mg twice daily in the aforementioned

European study; thus this dose, or a therapeutic equivalent dose of a longer-acting, once-daily ACE inhibitor, might be appropriate. An alternative would be to titrate the dose against the antiproteinuric effect of the ACE inhibitor.

Normotensive NIDDM patients with microalbuminuria

A majority of the trials involving the treatment of normotensive diabetic patients have focused on IDDM patients. However, a recent study by Ravid et al compared the effects of ACE inhibitor therapy (enalapril 10 mg daily) with placebo in normotensive NIDDM patients with microalbuminuria. Over a long follow-up period (five years) the ACE inhibitor therapy stabilised the albumin excretion rate, whereas in those patients receiving placebo therapy, there was a progressive increase in albumin excretion rate (Figure 33)[10]. The ACE inhibitor therapy also stabilised serum creatinine levels, whereas there was evidence of a progressive decline in renal function in those patients receiving placebo therapy. This study suggests that normotensive NIDDM patients with microalbuminuria may also experience protection against progressive renal injury with ACE inhibitor therapy. Whether there is also protection against CV disease, the major cause of mortality in this group of patients, awaits confirmation.

In conclusion, the use of ACE inhibitors to treat normotensive IDDM and NIDDM patients with persistent increases in urinary albumin excretion rate has emerged as a novel strategy to complement other approaches (improved metabolic control, etc.) in an attempt to reduce the increased renal and CV morbidity and mortality of these patients. The results of the published trials are very encouraging and have also served to remind us of the thoroughly depressing results of placebo therapy.

THE UNDERDIAGNOSIS AND UNDERTREATMENT OF HYPERTENSION IN DIABETES

Since the early 1970s it has been recognised that there is a significant under-diagnosis, undertreatment and inadequate treatment of hypertension in general. Studies from the UK and the US have demonstrated that, despite the high profile given to the need for screening and treatment of hypertension, half of all cases will remain undiagnosed. Of those diagnosed, only half will receive treatment and of those treated, only half will achieve adequate control of their blood pressure. This so-called 'rule of halves' (Figure 34) means that only 10-15% of all hypertensive patients will ever receive adequate medical care.

One might assume that the situation with regard to diabetic subjects with hypertension would be better than this, particularly in view of enormously high rates of CV disease and the high prevalence of hypertension in this

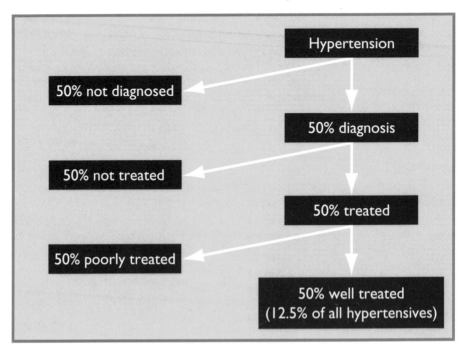

Figure 34 - 'Rule of halves'

population of patients. The recent report from the Hypertension in Diabetes Study Group[11], part of the UKPDS study, demonstrated that in a study of over 3,000 recently diagnosed NIDDM patients, over 39% were hypertensive (BP ≥160/90 mmHg). Of those hypertensive patients, 54% were untreated. In a further study[12], the prevalence of hypertension was examined in a large sample (5,842) of IDDM and NIDDM patients attending 10 diabetes clinics in and around London. As shown in Table 26, a very high percentage of IDDM and NIDDM patients with hypertension (BP ≥ 160/95 mmHg) were untreated. Moreover, of those on treatment, at least 35-40% still had unacceptably high blood pressure levels. When one considers the high treatment threshold for the diagnosis of hypertension in this study, it is clear that the undertreatment and inadequate treatment of hypertension in diabetic subjects is at least as common as has been documented for the general population, and probably worse when more stringent treatment thresholds are applied. Thus, even in this high-risk group, in whom great emphasis has been placed on the need for more aggressive treatment of hypertension, the quantity and quality of treatment appears to be inadequate.

The inadequacy of blood pressure control in those patients already on treatment is a particular cause for concern. It cannot be overemphasised that

Table 26 - The undertreatment and inadequate treatment of hypertension in diabetic subjects.	IDDM		NIDDM	
	Male	Female	Male	Female
% of diabetic subjects with hypertension receiving antihypertensive therapy	45%	34%	66%	69%
% of diabetic subjects receiving antihypertensive therapy but with inadequate blood pressure control	35%		40%	

the benefits of antihypertensive therapy are related to the quality of blood pressure control, i.e. the treated blood pressure level. Failure to achieve this therapeutic goal means that the patient receiving treatment holds an incorrect belief that the treatment is producing considerable benefit. Furthermore, the patient is exposed to the long-term side-effects of drug therapy. Moreover, the costs of inadequate treatment are enormous both for the patient and the health-care budget. It is likely that a major factor in the high frequency of inadequate blood pressure control relates to poor compliance with therapy or that hypertension is more resistant to treatment in patients with diabetes. Whatever the reason, these reports highlight an enormous opportunity missed and emphasise the need for careful screening programmes for hypertension in diabetic clinics, improved patient education regarding the benefits of antihypertensive therapy and continued clinical vigilance to ensure long-term and adequate control of blood pressure.

CONCLUDING REMARKS

I hope this book has served to emphasise that hypertension is by far the most important risk factor for mortality in diabetic patients. Indeed, large epidemiological studies, such as those from Framingham, US, have repeatedly demonstrated that hypertension is the single most important risk factor for the development of all CV events among diabetic patients. All of the available data supports the notion that hypertension in diabetic patients should be actively screened for and vigorously treated. However, the full benefits of antihypertensive therapy will not be realised unless the overall and considerable CV risk burden of diabetic subjects is simultaneously addressed. With this in mind, non-pharmacological strategies are particularly relevant and important in this patient population.

For the pharmacological management of hypertension, a hierarchy of choice of drug therapy is often easy to establish for individual patients by reviewing their associated CV risk, their established target organ damage and any diabetic complications that may preclude the use of certain drugs. This should ultimately identify the most preferable and exclude the least preferable choice of therapy for each category of patient. The overall goal of therapy is to modify favourably or eliminate all CV risk factors. Diabetic patients should be made aware that regular monitoring and control of their blood pressure is at least as important as control of their blood sugar. The importance of achieving and maintaining adequate blood pressure control in IDDM and NIDDM patients cannot be overemphasised.

REFERENCES

1. Dahlöf B, Pennert K, Hansson L. Reversal of left ventricular hypertrophy in hypertensive patients. *Am J Hypertens* 1992; **5**: 95-110.

2. Cruickshank JM, Lewis J, Moore V, Dodd C. Reversibility of left ventricular hypertrophy by differing types of antihypertensive therapy. *J Hum Hypertens* 1992; **6**(2): 85-90.

3. Kasiske BL, Kalil RSN, Ma JZ, Minjen Liao, Keane WF. Effect of antihypertensive therapy on the kidney in patients with diabetes: a meta-regression analysis. *Ann Int Med* 1993; **118**: 129-38.

4. Böhlen L, de Courten M, Weidmann P. Comparative study of the effect of ACE inhibitors and other antihypertensive agents on proteinuria in diabetic patients. *Am J Hypertens* 1994; **7**: 84S-92S.

5. Slataper R, Vicknair N, Sadler R, Bakris GL. Comparative effects of different antihypertensive treatments on progression of diabetic renal disease. *Arch Intern Med* 1993; **152**: 973-80.

6. Lewis EJ, Hunsicker LG, Bain RP, Rohde RD, for the Collaborative Study Group. The effect of angiotensin-converting-enzyme inhibition on diabetic nephropathy. *N Engl J Med* 1993; **329**: 1456-62.

7. Lebovitz HE *et al.* Renal protective effects of enalapril in hypertensive NIDDM: role of baseline albuminuria. *Kidney Internat* 1994; **suppl 45**: S150-5.

8. Agardh C-D, Garcia-Puig J, Charbonnel B, Angelkort B, Barnett AH. Greater reduction of urinary albumin excretion in hypertensive type-II diabetic patients with incipient nephropathy by lisinopril than by nifedipine. *J Hum Hypertens* 1996; **10**: 185-92.

9. Viberti GC, Mogensen CE, Groop LC, Pauls JF, for the European Microalbuminuria Captopril Study Group. Effect of captopril on

progression to clinical proteinuria with insulin-dependent diabetes mellitus and microalbuminuria. *JAMA* 1994; **271**: 275-9.

10. Ravid M, Savin H, Jutrin I, Bental T, Katz B, Lishner M. Long-term stabilizing effect of angiotensin-converting enzyme inhibition on plasma creatinine and on proteinuria in normotensive type II diabetic patients. *Ann Int Med* 1993; **118**: 577-81.

11. The Hypertension in Diabetes Study Group. Hypertension in Diabetes Study (HDS): I. Prevalence of hypertension in newly presenting type 2 diabetic patients and the association with risk factors for cardiovascular and diabetic complications. *J Hypertens* 1993; **11**: 309-17.

12. Fuller JH, Stevens LK and the Diabetes Hypertension Study Group. Prevalence of hypertension among diabetic patients and its relation to vascular *J Hum Hypertens* 1991; **5**: 237-43.

INDEX

A

abdominal aortic aneurysm 107, 139
Aborigines 64
absent foot pulses 139
ACE (angiotensin converting
  enzyme) inhibition 30, 81, 106,
  109, 115, 118, 121–123, 125–128,
  129, 131–147
acromegaly 37, 109
adrenaline 30
Afro-Caribbeans 19–21, 116, 119,
  122, 139, 144
age 16–21, 24, 31–32, 35, 37, 45–46,
  48, 51, 58, 64, 116, 135–136, 138
albumin excretion 24–25, 78, 142,
  146–147
albumin:creatinine ratio (ACR) 83
albuminuria 143
alcohol 32, 105, 113
aldosterone 30, 109, 125
alpha$_1$-blockers 115, 120–122,
  130–135, 139–140
ambulatory blood pressure
  monitoring 26–27
amiloride 127, 144
amlodipine 123, 124
angina 119, 123, 125, 133, 134, 135,
  138
angioplasty 47
angiotensin-I (AI) 30, 125
angiotensin-II (AII) 30, 121, 125, 129
anorectic drugs 106
anthropometric measurements 65,
  71
antihypertensive therapy 18, 38, 55,
  57, 72, 100, 103, 105, 112–147
antinatriuresis 35
antiproteinuric effect 140–141
aortic coarctation 37, 106
arrhythmias 107, 108
arterial blood pressure 16
arterial foot ulceration 51

arterial hypertension 48, 81
Asians 19–20, 64, 70–72, 74, 122
atenolol 143
atheromatous vascular disease 38
atherosclerosis 44, 47, 51, 68, 69–70,
  93, 106
atrial natriuretic peptide levels 30
atrioventricular nodal conduction
  123
autonomic neuropathy 115, 122,
  124, 127, 135

B

bedside diagnostic tests 83
bendrofluazide 116
benzothiazepines 123
beta-blockers 72, 106, 115, 117–120,
  121, 128–130, 132–133, 134,
  138–140
blindness 54, 88
blood clotting 67, 68, 94
blood flow autoregulation 52–53, 58,
  60
blood pressure
  control 148–150
  diurnal variation 27, 41
  measurement 104, 110
  thresholds 102–103
body fat distribution 106
body mass index (BMI) 16, 19, 32,
  64, 71
body weight 113
bradykinins 125
brain infarct 46
British Hypertension Society (BHS)
  101–102, 131
bumetanide 138

C

calcium antagonists 115, 121,
  122–125, 129–130, 131–141,
  144–145

calorie intake 113
captopril 109, 126, 136, 142, 143, 146
captopril renogram 109
carbenoxolone 106
carbohydrate metabolism 113, 117
cardiac
   death 49, 117, 137
   failure 45–47, 108, 112, 124, 126
   function 89–90
   myocytes 121
   murmurs 107–108
   output 36
cardiomegaly 108
cardiomyopathy 44, 60, 89–90
cardiovascular (CV) death 12, 65, 145
cardiovascular (CV) disease 12,
   44–49, 58, 60, 62–74, 76, 79, 84,
   86–87, 90–93, 97, 100, 105, 114,
   122, 139, 142, 147
cardiovascular (CV) risk factors 58,
   62–74, 94, 95, 101–103, 112–115,
   120, 130, 149–150
carotid artery stenosis 53
carotid bruits 106, 139
catecholamine levels 30–31
cell contraction 122
cerebrovascular disease 50, 60, 130
chest X-ray 108
chlorthalidone 116
cholesterol 67, 108, 117–118, 121,
   129
chronic open-angle glaucoma 55
cigarette smoking 46–47, 51, 56, 58,
   64, 85, 105, 114, 138
circulatory haemodynamics 35
claudication 44–47, 51
clonidine hydrochloride 128, 133,
   136–137
clot lysis 67, 68
clotting abnormalities 94
cold cures 106
cold hands and feet 130

combination therapy 131–132
congestive cardiac failure (CCF)
   48–49, 138
constipation 124
coronary heart disease (CHD)
   45–49, 60, 67, 114, 126, 137
coughing 127, 129–130
creatinine 108, 133, 139, 142–143
Cushing's syndrome 36–37, 106–107,
   109
CVA/TIA 44–45

D
deletion polymorphism (DD) 81
Diabetes and Hypertension Study
   Group 17
Diabetes Control and Complications
   Trial (DCCT) 12, 85
diabetes
   cardiomyopathy 49, 52, 138
   cardiovascular risk factors 58,
      62–74, 94–95, 101–103, 112–115,
      120, 130, 149–150
   hypertension 12, 16–21, 44–60,
      100–110, 112–150
   nephropathy 20, 24, 26, 28, 29, 32,
      36, 37, 39, 41, 44, 52, 53, 57–58, 60,
      68, 76–97, 112, 127, 134, 139–140,
      146
   neuropathy 44, 52, 56–57, 60, 84,
      89, 107, 112, 135
   pathogenesis of hypertension
      24–41
   retinopathy 44, 52–56, 60, 76, 84,
      87–89, 105, 107, 112, 130
dialysis 78, 80, 143
diastolic blood pressure (DBP) 16,
   25, 50, 55, 85, 102–104
diet 105, 113–114, 136
dihydropyridines 123–125, 140–141
diltiazem 123, 124, 138, 141, 143
dipstick urinalysis 108

diuretic therapy 121, 127, 136–137, 140, 144
diurnal blood pressure variation 27, 41
doxazosin 120, 122
drug therapy 105, 110, 115–147
dyslipidaemia 36, 56, 62, 65–66, 68, 74, 108, 112, 114, 117, 120–122, 134–135, 142
dyspnoea 130

E

elastic hosiery 136
elderly patients 116, 119
electrocardiography (ECG) 108
electrolytes 108
enalapril 126, 145, 147
endocrine causes of diabetic hypertension 37
endothelial dysfunction 31, 33, 94
endothelins 31
energy intake 113
enzyme-linked immunosorbent assays 83
epidemiology of hypertension in diabetes 16–21
ethnicity 16, 19–21, 64, 70–72, 74, 116, 119, 122, 139, 144
euglycaemic clamp 62
European Dialysis and Transplantation Registry 80
exchangeable sodium 25, 28–29, 33–34, 41
exercise 24, 27, 64, 74, 94, 105, 113, 120, 134

F

fat intake 113
females 17
femoral bruits 106, 139
fibre intake 113
fibrinogen 62, 68, 94
fibrinolysis 62, 67–68

fibrosis 19, 49
first-dose hypotension 122, 127
fludrocortisone 136
fluid retention 25
flushing 130
follow-up of treatment 131
Framingham Heart Study 45–48, 50, 63, 70, 149
frusemide 138, 143–144

G

gangrene 44, 51
gender 16, 17, 19, 47–48, 50–51, 56, 58, 65, 105, 127, 134, 137, 138
genetic factors 81
glaucoma 55
glomerular filtration rate (GFR) 78, 79, 143
glomerulosclerosis 25, 76
glucose 31–33, 35, 39, 41, 49–50, 62–63, 65, 69, 71, 100, 117, 119, 122, 124, 129, 133, 134
glycaemia 12–13, 68, 81, 85, 95, 105, 108, 112, 115, 150
glycated haemoglobin A1c 108
glycoproteins 49
glycosylation 66, 70
gout 130

H

haematuria 107
HDL cholesterol 56, 65–66, 71, 74, 108, 117, 119, 120, 121, 129, 134
headache 130
height 106
hydralazine 128, 138
hyperaldosteronism 28, 107, 109
hypercholesterolaemia 46
hyperfiltration 78
hyperglycaemia 54, 56, 62, 68–70, 74
hyperinsulinaemia 35–36, 39, 62–64, 66, 69, 71

hyperkalaemia 127, 133, 144
hyperlipidaemia 31, 65, 106
Hypertension Detection and Follow-up Program (HDFP) 100
Hypertension in Diabetes Study Group 148
hypertension
  evaluation of diabetic 100–110
  in diabetes 12, 16–21, 44–60
  management guidelines 101–103
  pathogenesis of in diabetes 24–41
  treatment 112–150
  underdiagnosis 147–149
  undertreatment 147–149
hypertriglyceridaemia 65, 74
hypoglycaemia 115, 119, 133
hypokalaemia 107, 108, 116–117
hyporeninaemic hypoaldosteronism 133, 144

I

IDDM (insulin-dependent diabetes mellitus) patients
  ACE inhibition 125–128
  alpha$_1$-blockers 120–122
  calcium antagonists 122–125
  cardiovascular injury 45–46
  cholesterol 66
  epidemiology 16–21
  evaluation of hypertension 100–110
  fibrinogen 68
  lipoprotein 68
  microalbuminuria 82–95, 142–144, 146–147
  nephropathy 57–58, 76–81
  neuropathy 56, 89
  non-pharmacological treatment 112–115
  pathogenesis 24, 27–31, 36–41, 113
  pharmacological treatment 115–147
  retinopathy 54–56
  underdiagnosis 147–149

Von Willebrand factor 68
immunoturbidimetric assays 83
impaired ejaculation 137
impotence 115, 117–119, 121, 123, 127, 128, 130, 133, 137
indapamide 118
insertion polymorphism (II) 81
insulin
  insulin:glucose ratio 62
  insulin-induced vascular growth 36
  insulin-mediated glucose disposal 63–64
  insulin-stimulated sympathetic nervous system activation 35
  resistance 35–36, 39, 62–66, 69–71, 72, 74, 94, 120–121, 126, 134
  sensitivity 112–114, 120–121, 126, 129, 135
  therapy 44
International Diabetes Foundation 104
interstitial fibrosis 49
interstitial oedema 28
intrinsic sympathomimetic activity (ISA) 119
ischaemia 44, 47
ischaemic heart disease 71, 93, 115, 119–120, 130, 135, 138
ischaemic optic atrophy 55
ischaemic optic neuropathy 55
ischaemic stroke 114
isolated systolic hypertension (ISH) 18, 20, 21, 36–37, 135–136
isosorbide dinitrate 138

J

Joslin Clinic Boston 16

K

Keen, Professor Harry 3, 82, 101
kidney basement membrane thickening 76
Kimmelstein-Wilson lesion 76

kininases 125
Krolewski 81

L
lacidipine 123
large vessel atheromatous disease 134
LDL 66, 108, 117
left ventricular hypertrophy (LVH) 27, 46, 49–50, 62, 74, 94–95, 107, 112, 119, 123, 126, 130, 133–135, 137–138
left ventricular mass index 50
lethargy 130
libido 137
lifestyle changes 130–131, 134
lipid abnormalities 58, 94
lipid metabolism 121, 122
lipid profiles 117, 120, 124
lipoprotein (a) (Lp[a]) 68–69, 94, 108
liquorice 106
lisinopril 126, 143
London Diabetes Hypertension Study Group 16
loop diuretics 133, 138, 144
losartan 129
Lundbaek, Knud 45
lupus reaction 128

M
macroalbuminuria 89
macromolecules 94
macrovascular disease 44, 47, 76, 90, 103, 112
macular oedema 55
maculopathy 55
malignant hypertension 39
men 17, 48, 50, 51, 56, 137, 138
mesangial matrix expansion 76
metabolic profile 44, 56, 60, 73, 117–118, 134, 142, 147

metabolites 109
methyldopa 128, 133, 136–137
Micral-test 83
microalbumin excretion rate 108
Microalbuminuria Collaborative Study Group 85
microalbuminuria 24–27, 29, 36, 41, 58, 68, 76–97, 125, 127, 133–135, 139, 140–142, 144–147
microangiopathy 51–53, 86
microvascular disease 12, 44, 51–53, 56, 68, 76, 90, 97, 103, 112, 142
minoxidil 128
Multinational Study of Vascular Disease in Diabetics (MSVDD) 58
Multiple Risk-Factor Intervention Trial (MRFIT) 67
murmurs 107–108
myocardial fibrosis 49
myocardial hypertrophy 49, 125
myocardial infarction 47, 67–68, 72, 79, 100, 112, 119, 123, 126, 131
myocardium 52

N
nephropathy 20, 24, 26, 28–29, 32, 36–37, 39, 41, 44, 52–53, 57–58, 60, 68, 76–97, 112, 127–128, 131, 139–140, 143
neuropathy 44, 52, 56–57, 60, 84, 89, 107, 112, 124, 135
NIDDM (non-insulin-dependent diabetes) patients
  ACE inhibition 125–128
  alpha$_1$-blockers 120–122
  calcium antagonists 122–125
  cardiovascular injury 45–46, 113
  epidemiology 16–21
  evaluation of hypertension 100–110
  fibrinogen 68
  fibrinolysis 67
  insulin resistance 62–68, 70–72

left ventricular hypertrophy 50
microalbuminuria 82–95
nephropathy 57–58, 76–81
neuropathy 56, 89
non-pharmacological treatment
112–115
retinopathy 54
pathogenesis 24, 28, 32–39
pharmacological treatment
115–147
underdiagnosis 147–149
von Willebrand factor 68
nifedipine 123, 136, 140–141
nitric oxide 31
nocturnal fall in blood pressure 36
non-diabetic renal disease 37
non-dihydropyridines 123–125, 132,
138, 141, 144
non-pharmacological treatment 74,
110, 112–115, 130, 134, 149
non-Q-wave myocardial infarction
123, 138
non-steroidal anti-inflammatory
drugs (NSAIDS) 106
noradrenaline 30
normoalbuminuria 24–27
Nycocard U-Albumin test 83

O

obesity 16, 24, 33–35, 37, 39, 41, 62,
64, 66, 71, 74, 105–107, 113–114,
120, 134
oedema 55, 107, 124, 130
optic nerve 55
oral contraceptives 105
oral corticosteroids 105
organ damage 27, 54, 82, 84, 95, 97,
103–106, 114–115, 130–131, 150
orgasmic dysfunction 137
orthostatic hypotension 104, 115,
122, 128, 133, 136
oxidation 66

P

palpitations 128
paroxysmal tachycardia 107
pathogenesis of hypertension in
diabetes 24–41
peripheral oedema 107
peripheral pulses 106
peripheral vascular disease 45, 47,
49, 51, 60, 69, 82, 92–93, 112, 115,
119, 133
peripheral vascular resistance 36,
118, 120, 123
perivascular fibrosis 49
PGH2 31
phaeochromocytoma 36–37, 107, 109
pharmacological treatment 74,
115–147
phenylalkylamines 122
physical exercise 24, 27, 64, 74, 94,
105, 113, 120, 134'
pigmented striae 107
plasma cholesterol 66–67, 122, 129
plasma concentrations 29
plasma fibrinogen levels 94
plasma insulin 35, 69. 70
plasma lipids 118, 120, 121, 122
plasma renin activity (PRA) 28–29,
33, 109, 118
plasminogen activator inhibitor-1
(PAI-1) 67–68
platelet function 67–68, 94
platelet-derived growth factor
(PDGF) 67–68
polycystic kidneys 107
polymorphism 81
post-myocardial infarction 128, 133,
135, 138
post-prandial glucose disposal 35
postural hypotension 122, 124, 130,
135, 136
potassium 117–118, 127, 139, 144
prazosin 120

premenopausal years 19, 47
pressor stimuli 27, 31
Prima Indians 64
primary hyperaldosteronism 37
proliferative retinopathy 87–88
prostacyclin 31
prostatic enlargement 107
prostatic outflow obstruction 121
proteinuria 17, 24, 29–30, 57–58, 68,
  76–97, 107–108, 124, 125, 128–130,
  133–134, 139–142, 144–146
pulmonary oedema 107

R

radio-femoral delay 106
radio-immunoassays 83
radioisotopes 109
radionucleotide cardiac imaging 90
ramipril 126
random growth hormone level 109
red blood cell/lithium
  countertransport 81
renal
  artery stenosis 38, 41, 53, 109,
    127, 138–139
  basement membrane thickening 76
  biopsy 76
  bruits 107, 139
  disease 16, 19, 24, 57, 68, 76, 84,
    93, 97, 105, 109, 115, 139–140, 142,
    144
  failure 78, 80, 86–87
  function 58, 76–77, 125, 128, 135,
    139, 143, 145, 147
  glomeruli 52, 78
  haemodynamics 141
  renin-angiotensin system (RAS)
    29–30, 125
  replacement therapy 78, 80
  sodium excretion 35
  ultrasound 109
renovascular bruits 139

renovascular disease 36–38, 107,
  109, 125, 128, 134–135, 138, 139, 146
renovascular stenosis 139
rest pain 51
retinal exudates 54
retinal perfusion pressure 55
retinopathy 44, 52–56, 60, 76, 84,
  87–89, 105, 112, 130
rule of halves 147–148

S

salt intake 113
screening for microalbuminuria
  83–84
secondary hypertension 41, 107–109
serum cholesterol 46
serum creatinine 78, 143, 144, 147
serum lipids 119
serum urea 139
side-effects of antihypertensive
  therapy 129–130
smoking 46–47, 51, 56, 58, 64, 85,
  105, 114, 138
sodium exchange 25, 28–30, 33–34,
  41, 116
sodium retention 28–31, 33, 35–36,
  117, 128, 133, 136, 144
spironolactone 127, 144
St Vincent Declaration Action
  Programme 83
stroke 49–51, 71, 100, 112, 114, 135
sudden cardiac death 49, 117, 137
supine hypertension 136
sweating 107
sympathetic nervous system
  activation 39, 120, 124
sympatholytic agents 128, 136–137
systemic hypertension 58
systolic blood pressure (SBP) 16,
  18, 25, 34, 46, 48, 50, 51, 55, 85,
  102–103, 113
Systolic Hypertension in the Elderly

Program (SHEP) 100

T
tachycardia 128
tachyphylaxis 120
target organ damage 27, 54, 82, 84,
  95, 97, 103–106, 108, 114–115,
  130–131, 150
terazosin 120, 122
thiazide diuretics 72, 100, 106,
  115–118, 121, 129–130, 132–134,
  138, 141, 144
thrombosis 44
thyrotoxicosis 36–37
timed urine sample 83–84
tissue plasminogen response 94
transplantation of kidney 78, 80
Treatment of Mild Hypertension
  Study (TOMHS) 121
triglycerides 65, 71, 108, 117–118,
  119, 120, 121, 129

U
underdiagnosis of hypertension
  147–149
undertreatment of hypertension
  147–149
United Kingdom Prospective
  Diabetes Study (UKPDS) 17–19
urea 108
urinary albumin excretion rate
  (UAER) 24, 26, 29, 30, 76–77,
  82–94, 107, 143, 146–147
urinary catecholamines 109
urine albumin:creatinine ratio 108
urine dipstick analysis 24, 77
USA Working Party on Hypertension

in Diabetes 101–102

V
vaginal lubrication 137
vascular
  ageing process 18, 37, 135
  endothelium 31
  hypertrophy 36
  injury 44
  toxin 70
  wall:lumen ratio 31
vasoconstrictors 31
vasodilatation 31, 106, 120, 123, 125,
  128, 135, 136, 137, 138
vasovasorum of peripheral nervous
  tissue 52
ventricular tachyarrhythmias 119
verapamil 123–124, 138, 141
Viberti 81
visceral fat 64, 66
VLDL cholesterol 117
Von Willebrand factor (factor VIII)
  68–69, 94

W
waist:hip ratio (WHR) 65, 71–72, 74, 106
water retention 128, 144
weight 74, 106, 113–114, 119–120, 134
Westernisation 64, 70–72, 74
women 19, 47–48, 50–51, 105, 127,
  134, 137
World Health Organisation (WHO)
  17, 58, 101–102

Z
zofenopril 126